Never Stop Healing

The Unknown Shortcuts with Peptides for an Extraordinary Life

Regan Archibald, Lac, FMP
&
Anne Markt

Never Stop Healing

Independently Published

Published in the United States of America

210825-01941.1

ISBN: 9798756083972

This book is not intended as a substitute for the medical advice of physicians. The reader should consult a physician in matters relating to his/her health and particularly with respect to any symptoms that may require diagnosis or medical attention.

For more information on 90-Minute Books including finding out how you can publish your own book, visit 90minutebooks.com or call (863) 318-0464.

Here's What's Inside...

Foreword

Hi, my name is Anne Markt. I co-authored this book with Regan Archibald, who is a friend and mentor I look up to. I've always loved writing and have dreamed of writing a book someday.

As I've learned more and more about personal growth and development over the years, I realized that "someday" will never come unless I actually start writing the dang book. I knew I had a lot to share, but did it matter? Would it make a difference for others?

When it dawned on me that now was the time to get started, I decided to ask Regan if I could practice my book writing skills by being his ghost writer. I didn't know what to write on my own, but I know Regan is a content-creating genius. I felt I could offer support for his upcoming book and potentially spur my own creativity in the process.

In true Regan fashion, he replied, "Why be my ghost writer when you could co-author the book WITH me?" He instantly validated my voice, the desire within me to share my own thoughts, opinions, and knowledge alongside his own.

That was the moment I realized the book I needed to write was this one. Making our online Group Coaching experience accessible in written form to share with the masses was a must. Did it matter? Absolutely. Would it accomplish the goal of making health transformation affordable and accessible? You bet! Did it give a place of meaning for me to share health stories so that people feel inspired, motivated, understood, and less alone? 100%!!

I also loved that it offered another learning format for those who prefer written over audio and visual learning. It would even offer our hearing-impaired clients a much easier way to study and absorb material, so here I am! I'm so honored and grateful to be a co-author on the first book (of hopefully many) in my life!

Here's a little about me and many stories to come as I believe stories are one of the most powerful communication tools we have. I majored in Musical Theatre at my dream school, The University of Michigan, Ann Arbor. Those were four of the best years of my life.

I graduated and moved to NYC, where I booked the off-Broadway show, *The Fantasticks*, followed by the Broadway National Tour of *HAIR*. I also performed in major regional theatres across the country, such as the St. Louis MUNY (largest outdoor theatre in North America seating 11,000), the Pittsburgh Civic Light Opera, and internationally in Tokyo, Japan. It was a wild, bumpy, beautiful ride. I'm grateful for every minute of it. I still sing on my own YouTube channel today. Check out www.annemarkt.com if you're curious.

While in college, I quickly learned the importance of learning how to take great care of my body to be able to perform. Unlike at a desk job, I couldn't just "phone it in" nor push through live shows if I caught every cold and flu. I also knew that Broadway performers looked vivacious, gorgeous and had to be at the top of their game to do eight shows per week.

I started seeing a dietician on campus for free, took a nutrition class as one of my academics, and read *SHAPE Magazine* articles religiously. Those three things ingrained in me how to count portions based on the FDA-approved food pyramid at the time, and how to count calories and macronutrients. My nutrition professor was obsessed with counting to the point of proudly telling our class he carries a scale with him to restaurants, so he doesn't go "over budget."

SHAPE Magazine, at the time, published articles about how dairy, whole grain wheat products, and other foods were great healthy options while also advertising things like Botox and other drugs on every other page. Yes, like you, I was taught from the get-go the importance of calories in, calories out, and low-fat foods.

As a result of this education, I grew to be obsessive, guilt-ridden, and developed body dysmorphia and binge eating from stress and a lack of understanding of how my body truly works. I'll never forget stepping on the scale after a workout years ago, having danced, lifted weights, run, and walked, all day, every day, and how deflated I felt when I saw I had gained weight (Not realizing I had gained healthy muscle mass and was in excellent shape!!). I also remember catching every single cold and flu that would go around campus because I didn't realize how stress, diet, and lack of sleep depleted my immune system.

Fast forward, and by the time I was 23, living in NYC as a full-time actress, I was stressed to the max. I would follow anything my western-trained doctors told me to do, even when my deeper instincts questioned it.

I continued to read *SHAPE Magazine* articles to learn about nutrition and push myself at the gym. If I gained weight, my go-to was calorie counting and restriction, going hard at the gym. Yes, I would lose weight until I found my appetite spinning out of control. I'd binge until I was in pain, feeling absolutely awful mentally and physically. Mix that with a neurotic mindset, and you have how my life felt in a nutshell. I was suffering in silence at the time. Being slim and saying you have a binge eating disorder wasn't believable.

When I first moved to NYC as a performer, I discovered by happy accident a school called the Institute for Integrative Nutrition. That led me to take their online course and become a Holistic Health Coach in 2013. I was done with not having real health knowledge and knew what I was doing wasn't working.

I discovered so much about myself in a year. I cut out gluten, dairy, soy, and corn, just to learn how my body responds to different foods upon reintroduction. I stopped calorie counting and stopped weighing myself. I learned how my cycle actually functions and that it has four phases (Thank you, Alissa Vitti, of Flo Living). Most women are NEVER taught that in grade school and beyond. We're taught that we have a "cycle" of about 28 to 32 days, and then we bleed.

That's about it. We learn nothing of the world in between and why we feel differently throughout the cycle. My lack of hormonal knowledge led me to believe my cycle would always be terrible, and I went on birth control for six years, ages 18–23, so I wouldn't have to deal with it.

The four phases finally explained why I didn't feel the same energy/emotions or appetite the first two weeks of my cycle compared to the last two. That level of understanding brought such compassion to my body's natural ebb and flow.

A couple of years after graduating, I decided I wanted to work with Functional Medicine Doctors who understood the importance of diet and lifestyle for their patients. Since that time, I've had the great fortune of supporting 12 Functional Medicine Clinics across the United States over the span of eight years.

I was a health coach, a manager, and a project manager. I spoke publicly as an advocate and brand ambassador. I acquired a lot of functional medicine and holistic health knowledge along the way, including biohacking (which is a world in and of itself).

I also became a meditator in 2014, learning The Ziva Technique by Emily Fletcher. That transformative practice helped me let go of binge eating for good, without even trying, something I had led myself to believe I might never overcome. Meditation also eliminated major motion sickness on plane rides which would sometimes leave me feeling vertigo for 24 hours on land or feeling debilitated from exhaustion after taking Dramamine to prevent it.

I've lost weight, and I've gained the weight back. I finally took the power back to learn and accepted that fad dieting and fad detoxing weren't choices I wanted for my life anymore. I no longer hate my body or weigh myself obsessively for a number to give me self-worth. I've taught women how to do the same.

If I could eradicate one major issue in the world (beyond cancer and preventable diseases), it would be body dysmorphia, eating disorders, and general mental illness. It causes immense psychological, emotional, spiritual, and physical suffering. When the mind is unwell and doesn't think well of the body, the body suffers as a result, and the vicious cycle continues. We put our bodies through intense workout regimens, diets, and burn out over and over to achieve an image like we see in movies and magazines.

It just doesn't work. My heart still breaks when I hear people I love or even complete strangers tearing apart their self-image and self-worth when, in reality, they simply don't understand WHY their body is responding and reacting that way, to begin with. If they had that knowledge and learned true self-worth and compassion, their lives would forever be transformed.

I'm here to tell you that if someone in your life is still telling you your health issues are simply a matter of calories in and calories out, please walk away. That's *not* your only solution. In understanding how your body functions and how your mindset affects your inner and outer world, you regain control and end the vicious cycle of self-inflicted suffering.

I've shared my story so that you understand that even the health-obsessed fall down and pick themselves back up again. My life is not a perfect shiny string of Instagram posts. I've struggled, and it's made me more resilient and a better coach, understanding the clients I work with on a deep, loving level.

Now, I'm not done on my own health and healing journey. As I write this, I still have things I am working on. I must constantly remind myself of all the things I've accomplished, as it's so easy to forget and discredit how far I've come. I'm nowhere near perfect, but that's an important facet of this book: *Never Stop Healing*. Health is a journey, not a destination.

I love this title Regan created because it reminds us all that we aren't seeking an end product to be reached. It's not a finish line. We are working on habit and behavioral change plus consistency, one day at a time, to achieve better and better results with time.

Once I stopped putting myself on fad diets every time a vacation or seasonal change or wedding was coming along, I got my freedom back. I choose instead to consistently do things that feel great and support me so that I look forward to events without using them as a reason to self-destruct.

A life of chronic anxiety, depression, and feeling "not good enough" is not the life any of us were meant to live. Why not try another way? A way in which you learn how to build healthy habits with simple foundational tools, get 1% better per day, and achieve greatness year after year. That's what Regan and I are here to teach you. We've seen it work, and we're here to share it with the world.

Get ready to have your mind blown by the knowledge Regan is about to drop on these simple yet transformative health techniques, and to realize your greatest potential in a much simpler, more practical format than you've probably ever experienced before.

We've had clients lose weight with breath work. We've had clients get their energy back on track with simple dietary shifts, 20-second cold showers, and proper hydration. This is the way of the future so that health is no longer something only accessible to the rich, famous, and few. This is how to *Never Stop Healing*.

Chapter One
A False Sense of Security

INTRODUCTION

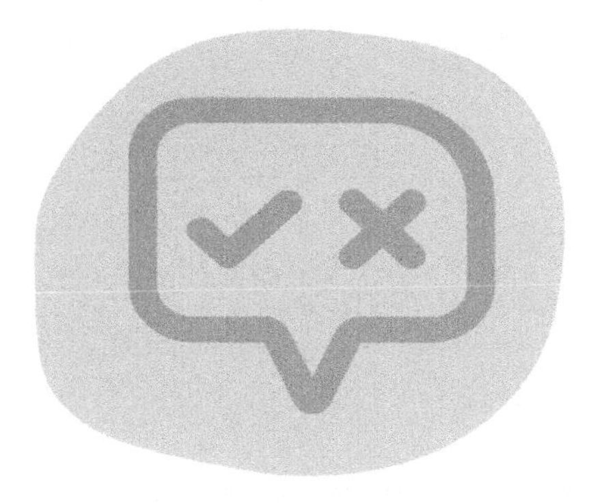

Your Health Can't Wait Until Tomorrow

Mindset Number One **My health and my life multiply when** **I invest in myself.**

This chapter will give you clarity on why it's time to create a higher standard of living for yourself. Feeling overwhelmed will keep you from making progress and what I promise to you is 100% clarity on the next steps in your journey to add life to your years and years to your life.

I see too many people struggling to grasp the reality of how their life is being impacted by their health. Now more than ever, we need to rise up to the greatness that is within each one of us by experiencing health at a new level. Now is the time to reflect on life's journey and discover the portal of health and greatness that's always been there because *your health can't wait until tomorrow.* A major event doesn't have to be what moves you into action.

Most people have no idea what great health feels like. We think that we have good energy and strength, and most of us dudes think we look a lot better than we do, or we justify our "dad bod" by saying to ourselves, "If I had as much time on my hands as he does, I would look like that too," and look down at our phone for a distraction from the discomfort we get from lying to ourselves.

We then laugh off the fact that we need to improve our diet, get to bed earlier and exercise by justifying the enormous joy that comes from watching the latest Netflix series with our favorite snacks, which we earned because we work hard and pay bills. "Every day, I'm Hustlin'," we rap to ourselves, not realizing that we are hustlin' *away* from the best version of ourselves.

A survey conducted by *Healthline* in 2020 found that 70% of Americans consider themselves healthy. This survey was taken by more than 2,000 participants who were asked about their work, sleep, and exercise habits, as well as their concerns regarding politics, the environment, and access to health care.

The average person slept 6.6 hours a day and exercised 6.9 hours per week, mostly walking. They also believed that they ate the right foods most of the time and had a healthy body mass index. "Take that, Regan! We are doing better than you've given us credit for!" Okay, okay, so maybe it's not that bad, but let's look a little deeper.

www.physiciansweekly.com/survey-most-americans-think-of-themselves-as-healthy/

A survey like this should make us feel pretty good, right? We think we are healthy, but unfortunately, it's not that simple. A 153,000-person study that was sponsored by the Centers for Disease Control (CDC) found that only 3% of Americans are living a healthy lifestyle.

What are the confines of a healthy lifestyle? The Mayo Clinic defines it as:

1. Moderate or vigorous exercise for at least 150 minutes a week (that's just 22 minutes a day).
2. A diet score in the top 40% on the Healthy Eating Index. (A government eating plan is hardly relevant after the failed science experiment called the food pyramid, but they have upgraded it some.)
3. A body fat percentage under 20% (for men) or 30% (for women).

4. Not smoking.
5. Alcohol in moderation.

This 2016 study found that only 3% *actually* meet these basic healthy lifestyle criteria, even though we are smoking less and making better food choices. This might come as a shock to you, but even in 2005, experts were finding that only 3% of people live healthy lifestyles. Since then, we've had a huge increase in information about wellness, yet we are still stuck in *preventable* chronic disease patterns.

I can tell you that, in my creation of the content for this book, I upped my game in my habits. I was able to gain 20 pounds of muscle, improve my testosterone levels, and increase my endurance in just 100 days! I was shocked at the results. I have some work to do because I started my practice in 2004 with the intention to transform health for as many people as possible. I guess we all have some work to do when it comes to health.

www.ncbi.nlm.nih.gov/pmc/articles/

www.livescience.com/216-study-3-percent-americans-live-healthy-lifestyle

Another poll NPR conducted with Truven Health Analytics, which surveyed a nationally representative sample of 3,000 U.S. adults in May of 2016, asked the question: "How healthy would you consider your eating habits to be?" About 75% of respondents ranked their diets as good, very good, or excellent.

Even though 75% of us think we are doing well, very well, or excellent, the reality is that only 3% of us are meeting the very basic levels of a healthy lifestyle. I would say we have some work to do around getting to the truth.

My friend and world-leading communication expert, Michael Bernoff, says, "Average Sucks." When people read that on his T-shirts or see the title on the cover of his book, they respond with, "Yeah, man, average does suck!" Michael corrects them and says, "No, **your** average sucks. You can do better."

There's a major disconnect in our society when it comes to health. We can all do better than our current "average." How many of you would put your life savings into an investment that had a 3% chance of having a positive return? That's the average!

Health is an investment, but we are putting our most valuable resource in a very risky position. We've been fooling ourselves into thinking that we are healthier than we really are, and in turn, we are putting everything on the line. Once you've had a heart attack or cancer or have been diagnosed with diabetes, you can't take back the years spent living a sub-optimal lifestyle.

You can do something about it ***now.***

www.npr.org/sections/thesalt/75-percent-of-americans-say-they-eat-healthy-despite-evidence-to-the-contrary

Want to add an extra seven years to your life?

Data gathered in 2017 by the Health, and Retirement Study found that people 50 and older who were normal weight, had never smoked, and drank alcohol in moderation lived on average **seven years longer.**

A 2012 mega-analysis of 15 international studies, which included more than 500,000 participants, found that over half of premature deaths were due to unhealthy lifestyle factors such as poor diet, inactivity, obesity, excessive alcohol intake, and smoking. The list of supporting research goes on.

www.healthaffairs.org/

www.sciencedirect.com/science/article

In this book, you will learn about brand new peptide therapies like Epitalon that enhance longevity. Most of you have already made a choice to live a healthy lifestyle, and I will introduce you to some incredible peptides that will turn on genes that express health and vitality.

Pause your reading and take a moment to breathe in deeply and slowly. Silence your thoughts as best you can and notice any sensations in your body. Do you feel that? The deep, calm reservoir of vitality in your lungs and belly? Do you sense the aliveness within?

As you feel the life within yourself, make the commitment to do everything you can to enhance it and create habits to support that feeling. Otherwise, your health will slip away. Today is all we can work with, so create some rituals in your life that will stoke the fire. It will pay off in ways you never expected.

Mindset Reset

What is going to be different about you in the next 100 days? Look in the mirror and ask yourself that question. How might your energy be different? What about your sense of wellbeing and confidence in your health?

Neuroscience tells us that your personality dictates your personal reality. What part of your personality will you change throughout this experience? The good news is that personality isn't permanent. (Thank you, Benjamin Hardy, and we highly recommend that book.) Thanks to neuroplasticity, you and your brain are far more malleable than you may think.

Take some time to set your goal(s) for this challenge of what you would like to see. Then take down some notes today so that you have trackable measurements of where you are now. Tracking and seeing your progress from beginning to end is a powerful accountability tool and reward mechanism in and of itself. There is no shame, judgment, or guilt.

Step one of any goal is to know your current baseline objectively. This also helps for awareness so you can constantly come back and see how far you've come, and your brain can't convince you otherwise.

As Anne mentioned before, be sure to focus not only on the end result. Have a strong why statement for why the goal is so important to you. What is it going to do for your life and the lives of others you're closest to? What is the worst-case scenario if you don't work on this goal now?

Lastly, make sure that you are focused, most importantly on consistency with the daily habit challenges you are given. It's simply about doing these small daily habits and watching the results show up for you with time. Letting go of what the results "should" be will quiet the skeptic within and make you less likely to let go of the habit if you aren't seeing huge results in a short amount of time.

Let's also redirect the focus away from general weight loss. We know now it's not the ideal measurement of health. For example, muscle weighs more than fat, and muscle building is a great thing!

If your goal is numeric, then make it a S.M.A.R.T. goal: Specific, Measurable, Attainable, Realistic, and Timely. Then keep a log so that you see the progress over time. Using a tape measure (or simply "how your pants feel") over a scale is a better indicator you are becoming a fat-burning machine!

That's another habit-building tip for you: seeing your progression little by little is wonderful and will keep your motivation strong. Rather than focus daily on whether you've attained your goal of 50 pull-ups yet, focus instead on your daily wins.

Did you do five to 10 pushups today? Maybe you noticed that the five you did today were easier than the five you completed yesterday. That's huge! Celebrate that and write it down. That's positive reinforcement that will keep you going strong every single day.

Now that you have a clear vision for your goal, please write down three fears. This helps give you a window into your own subconscious drivers of your current behaviors and what could come up as a challenge or sabotage your desire to reach your goals.

Let's try an example. Say you want to feel strong and energetic. Why? Maybe you want to be able to keep up with your kids, play with them, and set a great example for them. That's wonderful.

Finally, for those of you who want an upgrade in your health, the peptides that you will learn about are absolutely life-transforming. Here's to the healthiest version of you. We are here for you.

3, 2, 1 Ready for Take-Off

Now that you know health can't wait until tomorrow, you are ready to jump in.

Welcome to my 100-Day Body Reset Challenge (Peptides included!). I have created challenges for Fat Burn, Energy Reset, Pain, Heart, and Brain Health and have seen tremendous results. Check out some of these testimonials:

> *"Thank you! I love this class!!!!"*
>
> *"Drinking a lot more water and lost about 15 lbs."*
>
> *"I am making better food choices and lowered my fasting glucose level by 80 points."*
>
> *"Increased energy, lost 40 lbs. over the last year, sleeping through the night."*
>
> *"Got sugar under control and lost 15 lbs."*
>
> *"Fasting in the evenings lost about 5 lbs. Going to bed earlier."*

"Lost 50 lbs, changed life significantly eating lifestyle. I'm so grateful for this program. I had tried so many different ones with not much change over time."

Are you excited to dive in? Before we begin, let's go over some rules of the road with our Health Coach Anne so that you get the most out of this 100-day experience!

Rule 1: Mindset Resets

These small 1% daily gains you'll be learning are not only transformative, but they help you relinquish resistance over why you might believe you "can't be healthy".

"It's too expensive to be healthy." How expensive is being sick? Most people believe that if they carry a decent health insurance policy, that they can count on being taken care of. Being healthy is more about proper thinking about health than it is expensive. You will see that the challenges will save you both time and money once you incorporate them into your life.

"It's too hard to be healthy." The majority of these challenges are made to be so easy; your brain can't help but say, "Oh, yes, I can do that!" At the same time, you need novelty and a healthy dose of challenge. We used the "Goldilocks" model and created a system that can be customized to suit you and feel "just right."

"It takes too much time to be healthy. I'd have to spend two hours at the gym every day." (That's not true at all and actually counter-productive.) The majority of our challenges can fit into your day with just 20 minutes or less.

What other excuses are you making to not get the healthy mind and body you crave? We're here to help you eliminate them one by one with mindset resets every step of the way.

The mind has an incredible impact on the body's ability to meet and exceed challenges. YOU are your biggest challenge and excuse. Stop for a moment and ask yourself, "What is truly getting in my way, underneath all the surface excuses I make for why I can't be healthy?"

More than likely, the root of your concerns is the result of fear, uncertainty due to excessive information overload, or maybe even a lack of understanding of how your body functions. Maybe you are still following old fad diet advice that "fat makes you fat" and "sugar is good for you". Word to the wise: *It's not.*

www.nytimes.com/2016/09/13/well/eat/how-the-sugar-industry-shifted-blame-to-fat

Maybe, as Michael Bernoff teaches in *Average Sucks*, you feel "just average". Your average is created by the environment and relationships you choose to engage in every single day, internally and externally. The only way out of this pattern is to raise your average. Create new friendships and reengineer your environment to be better than it is now.

The challenges in this book will elevate your average, stretch your comfort zone, and allow you to become the best version of yourself. Fully engaging in each of the challenges requires courage. It's no different than starting a new relationship or learning a new skill.

Whatever it might be, write down your fear(s) at the start of each challenge as you go. Share them with someone. If you were your own best friend, what would you say in response? Try reframing that into a positive affirmation or belief. Then ask yourself, "What am I most looking forward to on this journey?"

One of the most fascinating things I've learned about psychology is that, once you've learned new information, like the "fat makes you fat" craze that created sugar-laden food products making us increasingly diabetic, it's hard to "unlearn" that false information. This is true even if information changes and finally reveals the original study to be false!! (Which it did, finally.)

There are still so many people who, without proper nutrition guidelines, go to the store and don't know *how* to read food labels. They don't know which foods to eat and which to avoid. With all the diets available out there, they throw in the towel before even starting, saying, "It's too hard to weed through all this information! How am I to know what is truly 'right' for me?!"

I know the feeling. Even as a health coach with years of experience working with patients in functional medicine clinics and wellness centers, I understand that frustration on a very personal level. I have read through endless information on diets and constantly experimented on my own health. The last thing I want to do is put out yet another "diet book" that creates more frustration and less clarity.

That's why it was so important that I join forces with Regan in writing this book. The techniques you are about to learn are soundly backed with scientific evidence and have been put to the test by biohackers, Regan, me, and many patients.

We walk the talk with these techniques in our everyday lives so that you have real-life evidence from our personal stories and patient victories of implementation. We also help you overcome the most common hiccups and challenges along the way. No time is wasted reading and implementing any of these techniques because they are already proven to work. It's just making time to implement!

Take a moment and write down what has been lost in not having started to work on your health sooner. **This is so important, so do not skip this!** This is going to help you craft your why statement, which you will learn about shortly.

Ask yourself honestly (and have compassion; this isn't about shaming yourself!), "What have I lost the past X years by not taking the time to work on my health?" Better yet (because language is powerful), "What have I robbed myself of in the past by not handling my concerns in the moment?"

Maybe you've robbed yourself of the chance of an incredible sex drive, time spent doing physical activities that bring you joy, or time spent with loved ones on trips or being in the outdoors because your health always got in the way. Maybe you've lacked energy, had headaches or general aches and pains, and had to skip out on fun adventures.

If you start to cry or feel angry, that's welcome. All feelings are welcome. That means we are on the right track to hit the core of why NOW is the time to start working on your health, and not a day later.

Do not waste any more life contemplating, struggling with, waiting, wanting, hoping, and wishing to be healthy. Today's the day to embrace a fresh mindset, tell yourself, "Yes, I can," and get started. No excuse is worth trashing your precious time and energy left on this earth.

Regan and I are here to take the stress out of the equation by showing you step-by-step, easy, affordable, time-efficient ways for how to boost your immune system function, energy levels, cognitive fitness, hormonal regulation, and so much more.

These are foundational tools that many (including myself) have taken for granted for years. The habits you'll be learning in this book are the "secrets" to success right under your nose, many of which have been used by ancient healers for centuries.

Are you ready to *finally* ditch the excuses and achieve the health you've wanted for years?

We are stoked to share this information with you in written format. Prior to this book, our Health Accelerator Challenges have been an online coaching experience offering daily accountability texts, weekly live lectures, and recorded 24/7 access to this incredible content. While that continues to be accessible to you, this written format expands our reach by giving people a learning tool that may better suit their style, especially for our hearing impaired clients or those who don't have great internet access. We want to further create a "no excuses" approach to getting you this valuable information for your health and wellbeing.

Rule 2: Have an Attitude of Gratitude

Oxytocin gets secreted when you do this! Positive psychology studies have proven the many benefits of just making a short list of what you are grateful for.

This is also important so that you don't lose track of all your wins along the way! Write down where you are at now and celebrate every single win, however small. It might be working up to 10 pushups a day or weaning off soda, or going from 10 seconds to 20 to 30 seconds of a cold shower! Celebrate it all!

I love this little manifestation tool. If you aren't where you currently want to be, start writing your gratitude lists and including the things you want, but in the present tense as if you already have them! Feel what that feels like.

Example: Say you want to feel greater energy. Write in a journal, "Today, I am grateful for my amazing energy!" You are slowly starting to rewire the brain and help it look for opportunities to fulfill that reality. Try it and do it consistently and see what happens!

Rule 3: Applied Learning

You must do these things to gain the benefits. Period. Just reading this book isn't going to make you healthier. Take these challenges seriously, and give yourself attainable goals that are S.M.A.R.T. (Specific, Measured, Attainable, Realistic, and Timely) so you know you are setting yourself up for success.

We have you start small with every habit, so each one is incredibly attainable. Writing down your baseline and tracking your progress on paper, in an app, or whatever metric works for you is ideal for the best outcome.

Rule 4: Accountability

Healing isn't meant to be done in isolation. What helps the brain learn new things is to go teach them to someone else. Not only do you benefit as you process the new information, but your friends and family do as well.

Ask your spouse to do the cold challenge with you. Tell your kids you are doing the "no sugar" challenge and make it a fun competition where whoever completes the challenge wins a fun prize.

You can even teach a co-worker how amazing you feel once you are properly hydrating and see who can be the first to hit their hydration goal for the day. Including those you love will make this experience that much more rewarding.

During the Protein, Fat, and Veggie challenge, plan your meals and eat with friends and family, share gratitude (per above) at the dinner table like Regan does with his family, and create a ritual of memories you will remember forever.

Rule 5: Make Every Challenge a Habit

This book is designed so that you go in the order we present the information. Each chapter will focus on one transformative habit from our Health Accelerator Courses. Regan will give you the science and research on why these habits are so vital to your health. Then my portions will be a mixture of health coaching, stories from my work with clients, stories from my life, and how to implement each habit using Habit Change 101.

Only do one habit every seven days! Make sure you feel solid with your implementation before moving on to the next habit. We still want you to continue the previous habit and stack them onto one another so that, by the end of the 100 days, you will have gotten 1% better every day and have achieved 100% results!

Along the way, you are going to be given "mindset reset" questions and challenged to know your own "why statement" behind each of these habits you embark on. Through years of studying habit change and personal growth and development from writers such as Charles Duhigg, James Clear, Simon Sinek, and others, I have seen the importance of starting with "Why" in anything I do. That coupled with "Identity Exercises" are, in my opinion, the two most underrated and overlooked elements of success when it comes to transforming your habits into what you want them to be.

Since I love habit change, I've laid out some valuable tools here for how to implement any habit into your life. I've learned from experience that my clients shame and blame themselves so deeply for not following through with instruction, rather than learning the primal tendencies of the brain and body and working in the flow rather than against it. You'll be able to use these tools as your foundation for any habit you wish to change for the rest of your life.

Each week, you'll read one chapter, then put the book down and immediately set your intention and game plan for implementing that One-Habit Challenge for the next seven days (and beyond). These habits are meant to be kept and followed long-term so that you see the benefits add up over time, like compound interest. The best part about this is that your only goal with these simple challenges is consistency. We've taken care of making it accessible (money, time, and ease).

While individual goals are encouraged and important for motivation, the focus is not on the end goals at all. It's in the process of consistency. That "one step at a time" and "one foot in front of the other" focus will help you stay on track so that you aren't focused solely on a number on the scale or expecting the results to come immediately.

Trust in the process, and with time, you will see exponential growth as these habits layer on top of one another and make you feel more alive than you have in years. (Have you ever caught yourself saying, "Wow, is time flying?" Use that to remind yourself how 100 days will be over in a flash, and you'll be 100% better with this implementation plan.)

What is Habit Building 101? Here's how to implement every one of our habits, as well as any "bonus" habits you want to accomplish in all areas of your life!

Step 1: Write down your Why Statement for completing this book and for doing these habit challenges. If you want to understand the power of "Why", watch this very short TED talk where Simon Sinek summarizes his theory. If you love it, I highly recommend his book to delve deeper: www.youtube.com/watch?v=u4ZoJKF_VuA

Why is your WHY so important? With any goal you set for yourself, there *will* be inevitable challenges that come up along the way, some harder than others. While we have kept things simple, we don't sugar coat it. Change, in the beginning before it becomes a habit, can be a challenge, and resistance can come up.

Your "Why Statement" is the statement you'll come back to that carries you through that resistance. It *has* to be extremely important to you (not just important to someone else). While you can absolutely create a statement that motivates you to do something for yourself that will positively impact someone else (a child, an elderly parent, a spouse, etc.), it must be something you can control and deeply meaningful and impactful for *you*. In fact, if it doesn't evoke some emotion within you, it's most likely not as strong as you'll need it to be.

Example: "I want to do these challenges because I want to lose weight" is not going to cut it. Throw the "I want to lose X lbs" out the window. It's totally fine for healthy weight loss to be a desire and a goal you wish to achieve. (If you read our testimonials, you'll see the common theme was that everyone saw weight loss!) We know the benefits of being a healthy weight, but your why statement behind that goal needs to be the deeper driver.

> *"I want to do these challenges because my weight is putting pressure on my joints and keeping me from being able to do the activities I love that bring me joy."*

> *"I want to do these challenges to correct my Thyroid concerns because if I don't handle this now using preventative techniques, I'll be setting myself up for dependency on medications or surgeries down the road. That will cost me more time, money, and stress, constantly having to manage my symptoms rather than eliminating the issue altogether. That would be like cutting a weed off in my garden without pulling its roots out of the dirt. I know it'll just keep coming back."*

> *"I want to do these challenges to boost my immune system and steer my body clear of cardiovascular disease, diabetes, obesity, cancer, and other issues that claim countless lives every single year. Why is that important?] I want to be around for my kids graduating, getting married, having babies, and all the most important moments of their lives and mine."*

What will your life look like 100 days from now?

What will bring a sense of progress and meaning to you?

What will life look like 100 days from now if you don't do anything or make any changes at all?

Be very specific about the changes you intend to see in the next hundred days. Be realistic and make sure that the goals are believable. Otherwise, you are setting yourself up for failure.

What are your top three fears heading into this challenge?

Fear can be a great motivator. So many of you have tried and failed, but this will be different. It's one day at a time. Lao Tzu said, "A journey of a thousand miles begins with a single step."

Keep in mind that if your why and your vision are too generic, it won't be strong enough to help you through those challenges when they come. Notice I said "when" not "if". Believing it will be a perfect steady upward progression is impractical and sets you up with the wrong mindset. Failure is part of the process. Just start again, and again, and again. Every successful person on the planet reached their goals because they were willing to push through their failures.

I know this works because once I learned the "Start with Why" model, I looked back and finally understood WHY some of my best efforts towards certain goals worked and why others didn't. When my goal was simply to "lose weight", it wasn't enough to get me to exercise in the dead of winter when the sun set at 4:30 pm in New York City. All I wanted to do in those moments was cuddle up inside my tiny warm apartment and say, "I'll do it tomorrow."

Once I changed the script and said, "I want to find an exercise routine that I absolutely LOVE so that I want to go consistently with far less mental resistance and feel awesome," it worked. The desire to go because I enjoyed it outweighed the inevitable moments I started to think about skipping. It no longer felt like a chore. That mental approach led me to find a gym I attended consistently four to five days a week for a year and a half, investing over $3,000 simply because I loved it! It wasn't about weight loss, and I ended up becoming stronger than I ever knew myself to be!

Step 2: Set your "Cue" or reminder. This is the first recommendation in the book *Atomic Habits* by James Clear, another must-read in the area of habit change. Your "Cue" is a pre-set device to trigger the brain and tell the body, "Do this now!"

Without that simple reminder, our brain and body (not having developed the habit yet) are far more likely to forget and continue on auto-pilot with the usual routines. That's why an easy way to start a new habit is to tack it onto the end of an already established habit to create a "When/Then" statement.

Example: "When I am making my morning coffee, then I'll put on my earpods and start listening to my binaural beats playlist."

That was the exact statement I created to implement the habit of listening to binaural beats every single day. Otherwise, even with the best of intentions, I noticed I kept forgetting throughout the day. Having my earpods next to my coffee maker "cued" me to start the habit.

Step 3: Make it appealing. While this isn't 100% necessary to implement a new habit or routine that is good for you (i.e., I don't believe many people *crave* brushing their teeth every day), there is still so much evidence to support the impact of this one element of habit building. Adding in the craving will maximize your consistency rate, especially in the beginning when you need it most.

You might be thinking, "Sure, Anne, but how am I supposed to crave something I don't like doing, even if I know it's good for me?" I get it, but this is where we switch the mindset and ask ourselves, "Is there a way I can adjust the environment to make this routine more attractive?"

Example: If you go through all the effort to prep your food for the week, make sure the presentation is attractive! If your food is wrapped up and stored in a way that's unappealing, you are far less likely to want to eat it than if it's chopped, vibrant, and ready to grab in your fridge!

More times than not, you have control over your environment and how you set it up. Make your habits obvious and attractive to get the motor running and trigger the routine itself. This brings us to our next step.

Step 4: K.I.S. = Keep It Simple. Life can be hard enough. Take control of what you CAN control and make these habits so easy to do; it's practically resistance/excuse-proof.

Here's an example. We will be teaching you the importance of cold exposure and its many health benefits. Before your brain makes you believe you have to buy some expensive cold plunge tub, invest in a biohacking membership, drive to the nearest lake or ocean, or sit in it uncomfortable for 10 minutes, simply start with doing ***20 seconds*** of your regular shower routine as cold water instead of hot.

That would be the time it takes to warm the shower up where you hop in without waiting, or you could warm yourself up and do it at the end. Sing *Happy Birthday* twice, and you're done. It costs $0, 0 extra time, and 0 extra effort to turn your shower handle!

Step 5: Make it fulfilling. Like making it appealing, this is often overlooked. Just like I've seen the effect of having a strong why statement on my ability to achieve certain goals, I've seen the power of making certain habits gratifying and how much more consistent I am at implementing them. I use my primal brain's natural tendency to my advantage.

What makes something worthwhile is different for each person. Just be sure the benefits are equally satisfying and beneficial, without being addictive or counterproductive.

Example: Please don't reward yourself for doing these habits with a chocolate binge or drinking wine or habits I call "win/lose". That causes you to win now (only in the present moment, and it's usually very, very short-lived) and lose later (feeling hungover, more tired, overly full, brain fog, etc.).

Instead, choose something visual that makes you proud! Mark your progress on a calendar you see daily. I like putting colorful star stickers on a calendar as it's both attractive and rewarding to see my progress that way. Yes, they are the kind you give to kindergarteners, but they cost me $5 on Amazon!

You could even make yourself a punch-card and ask your trainer or teacher to punch it each day you come so you are simultaneously reminded (Cued) to keep up the good work. Having a trainer or friend who knows your goals is another great accountability tool.

The beauty about all of these things is that you hold the power to implement each and every one of them. It's not about willpower. While you do have a finite amount, and you could push your way through anything, I believe life is not meant to be such a struggle bus.

Start using these techniques immediately, and you'll see for yourself. Start with something simple like, "I want to always know where my keys are," and make it a habit of storing them in a specific pocket of a purse or have a welcome stand by your door.

Those are the steps in a nutshell. Please review them often, and as mentioned, for an in-depth look into each of those recommendations, further examples, studies, and research, definitely check out *Atomic Habits* by James Clear and Charles Duhigg's *The Power of Habit*.

As long as you have your Why Statement completed for Why you are choosing to read and implement what is taught in this book, you are ready to dive into the next chapter.

Another free simple transformative tool to shift your energy, focus, and connection is to write a gratitude list every day. Keep tabs on your progress and your personal wins, and then come share them with us! We want to hear all about your successes and help you with your own personal challenges, whatever they may be so that nothing stands in your way.

If you are skeptical that these simple changes, 1% daily, can truly shift your health for the better, don't take our word for it. Review these incredible testimonials again from our patients who have gone through this exact same 100-Day Challenge!

> *"I'm drinking more water and have lost 15 lbs!"*
>
> *"I am making better food choices and lowered my blood glucose level by 80 points."*
>
> *"I have increased energy, have lost 40 lbs.* (in a year, this included)*, and am sleeping through the night."*
>
> *"I've eliminated plastics from my life as much as possible."*

My favorite from a patient who also did Peptides:

> *"I'm feeling Freaking GREAT!!!*
>
> *"I'm feeling much younger, much less fatigue, more energy, much less anxiety, more calm and clear in my thinking.*
>
> *"More stable blood sugar, better digestion and elimination, and a bit better with sleep."*

One client credited the Breath work you'll be learning in chapter 5 most of all for helping her to lose 20 lbs. in the course of the 100 Days! It all adds up.

Now that you are mentally primed and know your "Why Statement", know how to create habits, and how to HAC with success, let's get started with Challenge number 1!

P.S: You're going to notice at the end of each chapter is a recommended Peptide that will help you with each of these habits and your overall health exponentially. Peptides can be taken as supplements to support cellular communication. They've been transformative for our patients, so we wanted to share and start getting you familiar.

At the end of the book, you'll also find a Bonus chapter with all the recommended peptides listed throughout this book in one place. Contact Regan at regan@gowellness.com if you are interested in learning which peptides would be best for you.

Inner Genius

I'm someone who loves to find bypasses to feeling my best, especially when it comes to brain health. Over the past ten years, I've spent a considerable amount of time researching and experimenting with nootropics because of the impact they have on brain performance and health. They help improve memory, help with stress tolerance, and assist with focus. "Inner Genius" is a formula that I created which is a natural nootropic that will give you the edge needed to optimize your capabilities in this new phase of your life. You can find it at thesmartmedicine.com.

Chapter Two
Stress

STRESS

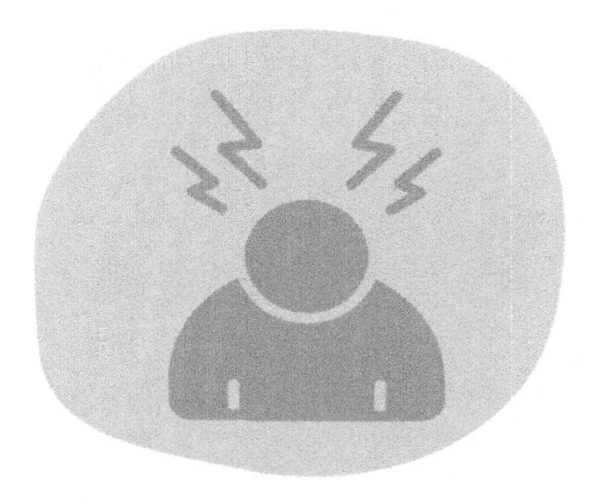

Vagal Tone Your Way to Relaxation

Mindset Number Two
An attitude of gratitude can change my entire body.

Answer this: What is your "happy place"? When do you feel in your best state of mind, body, and spirit, and what activities/environments get you there? Do you have a memory of when you have been the best version of yourself that you can anchor to, manifesting your greatest potential?

Examples could be being outside gardening, taking a hike, or enjoying nature. It could be connecting with your loved ones. It could be when you are "in the zone/flow-state" and lose track of time because what you are doing brings you so much joy! The sky's the limit! Please write yours down.

> *"Your sacred space is where you can find yourself over and over again."* ~Joseph Campbell

Your sacred space can be the perfect place to come back to time and time again to refresh and remind yourself what matters most to you, feeling "at home" and centered in your true self.

As you go about this book, there's another mindset that is very important to take note of, especially for my "Type A" personalities out there. If I could go back in time and talk about this in my first session with every client I have ever worked with, I would.

When it comes to your pursuit of a healthy lifestyle, be sure that your aim isn't for perfection. The mindset of "all or nothing" has been a top psychological distortion that has caused so many of my clients, including myself, to throw in the towel on a new habit or desired change only days, weeks, or even months after the onset. This is all due to a false belief that we have to be 100% perfect with changes or it wasn't "good enough".

As you go about this journey, we're going to start by aiming for 80% proficiency with each habit. Can you commit to something 80%? More likely than not, that alleviates pressure and brings about more feelings of positivity, calm, and confidence than if I were to ask you if you can be 100% perfect with all these habit challenges from the beginning.

As a coach, it would be foolhardy for me to ever ask that of a client. I know we are all human and bound to stumble and zig zag on the path, yet so often, we unconsciously expect this perfect level of fortitude from ourselves. Any wise therapist, mentor, or sage will tell you that embracing the inevitable highs and lows of a journey will bring far greater peace and even solutions than trying to avoid any problems or pitfalls.

I am a personal growth and development enthusiast and have been introduced to *so* many psychological perspectives in all the books that I've read and theories that I've come across. In that process, I've learned a very important lesson about myself as a human being that I think (and hope) will help you tremendously if you can relate to this as well.

In pursuit of happiness, success, excellence, and my best health and best self possible, I've often negated a part of me that has been and will always remain there in an effort to try and live a "perfect life". In reality, that approach has caused me a lot of unnecessary internal struggle that steals the available joys along the journey of self-actualization and fulfillment.

In the book, *The Upside of Your Dark Side* by Todd Kashidan and Robert Biswan-Diener, I was reminded of something that not many of the spiritual and personal growth and development books I've read talk much about. That's quite literally embracing a part of your human nature rather than rejecting it.

While 80% accuracy is a phenomenal place to start with regard to these goals, it still leaves that 20% to be managed. Considering the brain very much gravitates towards the negative, it can be easy to blow up that 20% inaccuracy and fill ourselves with regret, shame, blame, and other negative feelings, simultaneously forgetting about the 80% we are doing very well! (The brain can't focus on the positive and negative at once.)

Rather than ignore that part of ourselves, I want you to embrace it as a part of you that will always be present and can and does contribute to creating a "whole" version of you, as the book above describes. Imagine a life in which you don't reject a percentage of yourself but rather embrace, acknowledge, and work in conjunction with it, believing you have everything you need and are exactly where you need to be every step of the way. What images does that conjure up for you?

For me, someone who has struggled with perfectionistic tendencies and seen the younger, less mature version of me give up on things I couldn't be "perfect" at, it's a welcome relief! While there are many die-hard biohacking, nutrition, and fitness enthusiasts out there who may cringe at the idea of aiming for 80% to start, in actuality, it sets the stage for even greater accuracy and success at the start of the journey as well as every step of the way. As a fellow Health Coach friend once taught me, it's the "good, better, or best" choice in any given circumstance rather than good or bad.

For example, when I used to tell myself in my early 20s that I couldn't have an ounce of gluten or I was "cheating on my diet", causing myself harm, and/or a myriad of other negative emotions, guess what I wanted to eat most of all and what I felt most guilty for bingeing on? The brain wants what it's told it can't have.

Similarly, I've witnessed many friends and clients justify their mentality of "perfect" on weekdays and then "letting loose" and bingeing on junk on weekends. It's just another psychological tactic to avoid discomfort when making change. We're promoting lifestyle changes here, not a diet to adhere to for a condensed period of time.

After years of all-or-nothing thinking, I've reached a mindset with gluten where I do favor the benefits and health of the "future me", wanting to feel clear-minded, no bloat, and more energy for the next 24 to 72 hours rather than succumbing to temptation in the moment. Does that mean I'm always perfect? Nope! I do eat gluten on occasion (gasp!), but funny enough, with far less frequency than I used to when I told myself I had to adhere 100% all the time. Interesting paradox, don't you think?

In telling yourself to start with 80%, you are relaxing the brain, giving yourself room for growth and improvement, not aiming for perfection. You are far more likely to do things well above the 80% mark than if you had aimed higher from the start. With any new habit or goal that you set, it's best to always make it incredibly easy to get started so that your brain doesn't become overwhelmed and create every excuse for why you can't get started.

Along the way, I hope you start to learn to forgive any mishaps immediately and treat all of your health experiences as learning opportunities for further growth and wisdom. Embracing that perspective and self-talk will do you a world of good, accepting your whole self and not rejecting your 20%.

Now that your mindset is refreshed, and I've hopefully alleviated any lingering stress heading into these challenges, let's dive into the science of Stress, the Hormone Cascade, and Vagal Tone!

How does stress manifest?

Let's go through the myriad of hormones and chemicals that occur within the body from the moment we experience the start of a stressful situation.

When you receive sensory information, the amygdala gets triggered to go into fight or flight.

> *"The amygdala is a collection of cells near the base of the brain. There are two, one in each hemisphere or side of the brain. This is where emotions are given meaning, remembered, and attached to associations and responses to them. They are emotional memories.*

The amygdala is considered to be part of the brain's limbic system." ~Healthline, Medically reviewed by Timothy J. Legg, Ph.D., CRNP, Written by Nancy Moyer, M.D. on April 22, 2019

Once the amygdala gets triggered, the hypothalamus ("H" of the "HPA" Axis) turns off your "rest and digest" parasympathetic system, saying, "It's go time."

Corticotropin-Releasing Hormone kicks in, which stimulates your pituitary gland (the "P" of the HPA Axis). The pituitary gland produces Adrenocorticotropic Hormone. This tells your adrenals (the "A" of the HPA Axis) to produce more cortisol.

A Simple Way to Test your Adrenals. While sitting in a chair, bend your torso over your legs so that your head is dangling between your legs. Remain there for about 30 seconds. Then lift up quickly! If you feel dizzy/nauseous, that could be a sign your adrenals are shot.

If you walk up a flight of stairs and feel fatigued, you may have an adrenal issue.

Cortisol is an "Alpha" hormone of the body that affects everything downstream. It's an important hormone, not a bad one! We just want the right amount at the right times.

Example: Cortisol should be highest in the morning as it's meant to wake you up! It's then meant to taper off as the day progresses and be lowest at night so that melatonin takes the lead. (You'll see later on why this is so important for your circadian rhythm.)

If you were to do a salivary cortisol test, and you discovered low levels in the morning and higher levels at night, this could explain why you feel like you can't get out of bed in the morning, yet you are tired and wired in the evening when you want to crash.

This "HPA" Axis governs all hormones in the body. This is how your brain communicates to the pituitary and adrenals. If this is dysregulated, you'll have imbalances in hormones like estrogen, progesterone, testosterone, DHEA, pregnenolone, etc.

Here's what can happen and can be associated with chronic stress:

- Decreased Immune System function
- Decreased Metabolism
    - This can explain that stubborn weight that won't go away. Think of it like the body trying to protect itself like a pufferfish when it thinks it's in danger.
- Depression
- Hypertension
- Chronic Fatigue
- Sleep Deprivation
- Migraines
- Tunnel Vision
- Acid Reflux Disease/GERD
- Hostility
- Hunger
- Arthritis

Long term, this can lead to increased blood pressure and cholesterol. Next time you are at the doctor's office, if your BP or cholesterol is high, try to work on stress, diet, and lifestyle FIRST before jumping on a BP medication or statin. Many times that can do the trick before needing to be dependent on a drug that doesn't truly correct the underlying cause.

How does one balance their HPA axis?

One thing that governs everything, and has a profound effect on your nervous system, is the Vagus Nerve.

The Vagus Nerve serves as the body's "superhighway", carrying information between the brain and internal organs and controlling the body's response in times of rest and relaxation.

The vagus nerve originates in the brain and branches out in multiple directions through the neck and torso, where it's responsible for such actions as carrying sensory information from the skin of the ear, controlling muscles we use for swallowing and speech, and influencing the immune system.

The word "vagus" means wandering; hence it is known as the wandering nerve affecting so many different organs and processes in the body. It's one of the longest nerves in the body and connects the brain to the gut!

There are fewer nerve endings in the spine compared to the gut. Have you ever noticed that when you start to feel stressed, you feel it in your belly? Butterflies in the stomach, cramping, a "nervous/anxious" feeling in the stomach, pain, nausea, etc., we "feel" things taking place in the gut because it's all interconnected.

You want your vagus nerve to be toned and strong. A weak vagus nerve can lead to a worsened stress response and less of an ability to tap into rest and digest or parasympathetic mode.

Autonomic Nervous System

There are three main parts that make up what is called the Autonomic Nervous System in the body. Sympathetic (fight or flight), Parasympathetic (rest and digest), and Enteric (which governs the gastrointestinal tract). The autonomic nervous system is a control system that acts largely unconsciously and regulates bodily functions, such as heart rate, digestion, respiratory rate, pupillary response, urination, and sexual arousal. This system is the primary mechanism in control of the fight-or-flight response.

What happens when this fight or flight response activates? The body responds in kind by going into a heightened state with increased heart rate, bronchial tubes in the lungs dilate to take in more oxygen, muscles tense, and glycogen is converted into glucose (also known as gluconeogenesis).

This process helps us quickly get out of a dangerous situation, like running from an animal or fighting to defend ourselves. Have you ever heard of someone pulling a car off of someone as if they had superhuman strength? Leave it to fight/flight mode to get us hyper-focused on the task at hand and provide energy to get us through.

The danger is not in having this stress response. We need it to survive! However, when it doesn't turn off, we have a problem, especially with small triggers that are non-life-threatening but still create the stress response, such as a phone call, a text, an email, etc.

There may be signs to show when the Vagus nerve is damaged or not performing well. These include:

- Difficulty speaking or loss of voice
- A voice that is raspy/wheezing
- Trouble drinking liquids
- Loss of gag reflex
- Pain in the ear
- Unusual heart rate
- Abnormal blood pressure
- Decreased production of stomach acid
- Nausea or vomiting
- Abdominal pain or bloating
- Leaky gut
- Addictions
- Alzheimer's
- Migraines
- Anxiety
- Depression
- Poor blood circulation

- SIBO (Small Intestinal Bacterial Overgrowth)
- Gastroparesis
    - Lack of enzymes and lack of the wavelike motion needed to move food through the body, leaving you with nausea and bloating
    - Nutrient deficiencies can happen as a result
- Insulin resistance
- Circadian rhythm and sleep patterns being off track

As you can tell, so much is impacted, and so much depends upon a strong vagus nerve!

The good news is many of the things we are teaching in this book can strengthen your Vagal Tone:

- Deep breathing
- Hydration
- Cold exposure
- Gargling water
- Singing or humming
- Meditation
- Enzymes, probiotics, and omega-3s
- Exercise
- Yoga
- Massage
- Social time, fun, and belly laughs :)
- Sleep on your right side to help "drain the liver"!

- Devices can stimulate it as well, such as the Apollo Neuro. Apollo has vibration frequencies to choose from that help stimulate parasympathetic tone.
- Positive emotions (Think "finding your sacred space" as we described at the beginning of the chapter.)
- Acupuncture can also stimulate vagal function! A study has shown this to be more powerful than implanted VNS (Vagal Nerve Stimulation) devices! https://pubmed.ncbi.nlm.nih.gov/24359451
- Peptides like Melanotan and KPV can help activate and reset the HPA axis, along with BPC-157, which promotes blood vessel formation and transports nutrients, supporting damaged nerves and brain cells

A very interesting study was done on meditators who practice with others/feel socially connected vs. meditators who do so on their own without the positive emotions of social connection. Those who felt connected showed higher vagal tone, as measured by heart rate variability, compared to those who meditated solo. This is very important to note!
pubmed.ncbi.nlm.nih.gov/24585500

While we could write an entire book on this one topic, and many have, I hope you've enjoyed Regan's introduction to stress, hormones, and vagal tone.

When I first heard Regan provide this presentation on stress, it all resonated with me very deeply. Stress has played a major role in my health over the years and learning to manage it while understanding my body's natural processes has been key.

I've always focused on stress reduction, but there are many great tools to use when it comes to mental stressors above and beyond taking a bath and lighting aromatherapy candles (though both are great options).

Let's be honest: Nine out of ten times, when we are in the midst of a stress response, we can't do common relaxing activities. It's possible we are in public or even at work when the stress response occurs. Let's start with recognizing which bucket it falls into and then practical things to do for in-the-moment stress relief as well as prevention.

By the way, there's also something to be said for the fact that not all stress is "bad". How we perceive stress matters more than the stressful occurrence. Viewing stress as purely "bad" or believing we can't handle it will only amplify the stress. Using any stressor as a growth opportunity and believing you have the tools to manage it can make all the difference in the world.

Step 1: Awareness

Start by logging a "Food/Mood" Journal so you can begin to make connections to activities, foods, lifestyle choices, habits, conversations, etc. and how everything makes you feel emotionally, physically, and energetically. Include all the data in one place: sleep, water, exercise, food, mood, bowel movement(s), what day of your cycle you are on as a female (Day 1 is the start of your bleeding), any life events that have occurred such as changes in relationships, job/career, etc. The mood section includes any emotions you are feeling, by the way, not just stress.

This will come in handy in creating your baseline for all of these habits to come, and it will also come into play in "Optimizing your Gut" later in the book!

Also, when it comes to working with a Functional Medicine provider and Health Coach, the more data you provide, the better. I love helping people connect the dots and realize all the powerful shifts they can make to their daily habits that, many times, nip a lot of physical stressors in the bud fairly easily.

That being said, habit shifts take some time and patience, especially when mentally driven. Knowing where the stress is stemming from (mental, physical, or both) helps you to "meet the problem at the level of the problem" (or better yet, possibly realize there is no "problem" at all).

When it comes to physical stressors, every single one of these habits you are learning in this book will help. Boosting sleep quality reduces stress by day. Eliminating sugar reduces the stress and inflammation that consuming it causes to the body. Cold showers help the body adapt to stress and boost vagal tone. Exercise helps the body metabolize cortisol.

On the other hand, if it's a mental stressor, here are some helpful questions you can ask yourself to bring more clarity to the situation at hand:

1. What part of me feels triggered right now? Where might that be stemming from?

2. How do I feel? (All emotions welcome, be honest with yourself.) Name it, give it a measure on a scale of one to 10, 10 being the worst. You can even give it a color/shape if you'd like. That way, you can also measure how you feel after an activity, so you know if it's working and improving.

   Example: I feel angry; on a scale of 1 to 10, it's about a 6, and it feels like a red baseball-sized lump in my throat.

3. Do you have the option to avoid this situation entirely? This is a great technique for things you can control in your immediate environment that maybe you don't need so much of, like social media, triggering FOMO or jealousy, excessively reading the news and feeling anxious, reading emails too early or too late in the day and feeling frustrated/overwhelmed, working late in the evening and not setting healthy boundaries when you in need of some quality time at home or on vacation. You have a lot more power over your environmental choices than you may realize. You know your limits. Use this one wisely.

4. If you can't avoid the situation entirely, can you change certain parts of the situation that you do have control over?

   Great example: Going to family gatherings used to stress me out when I was a binge eater. I now look forward to shared food events because I know I can bring foods to share that I love that don't derail my desire to eat well. I bring plenty so others can learn how delicious healthy foods can be without feeling deprived. That created a new experience.

5. What if you can't avoid or change the circumstances at all? Maybe someone has passed away, or something someone else is doing at work is bothersome and can't be changed. A great tool for these moments is learning to "flip the script" and reframe your thoughts towards the person/place/thing/circumstance. Some great resources for this are <u>*The Work*</u> by Byron Katy, *The Artist's Way* by Julia Cameron, and a short easy course called *Procabulary* by Mark England.

   One of my favorite tools in Mark England's course is to take a statement such as, "Bob made me feel ______," which is a projection statement, then add, "and my only option is to feel _____." This tool alone starts getting the gears churning to think about what you do have control over in any given situation. You only have control of yourself and how you respond.

6. If none of the above options are working to the extent that you need them to, it's time to use a very powerful approach by teaching your body to adapt and better handle the myriad of stressors: de-stimulating the response so triggers no longer phase you and/or leveling up to meet the challenges at hand with greater ease.

   I like to refer to this as the "Mario gets a Mushroom" effect for you gamers out there. In the video game, *Super Mario*, when Mario gets a mushroom, he grows bigger and can tackle his opponents with greater ease. This is extremely beneficial for when life throws you curveballs, trauma, heartbreak, or major setbacks.

Start doing this now and do it every day! Adaptation exercises (to uplevel your consciousness) could be meditation, mindfulness exercises, exploring your spiritual side, Emotional Freedom Tapping, and other physical or mental techniques that help you see the greater picture.

Don't wait until the stressors *come* to do these actions. Having these consistently in your routine and in your system will help eliminate/avoid triggers that used to send you flying. It's like taking your mind to the gym using an activity. Doing some physical activity when emotion/stress feels high is one of the best things you can do. If you can take a walk, go for a run, or if yoga is your haven, do what works for you.

Above and beyond the options above, having a support system like a therapist, mentor, and/or coach to help you reframe and give you space to talk things out is extremely beneficial. We highly recommend that alongside all the work you are doing for your well-being.

Stressors Come in Many Forms and Vary for Everyone. They could come in the form of family demands, relationship (communication issues), maybe working towards a degree or certification, workload, work-life balance, emotional triggers, and pain. Even the emails, texts, and social media we feed our brains excessively on a daily basis can send the body into fight-or-flight mode without us even realizing it!

Pretty much all of those stressors fall into one of four main categories: Emotional, Mental, Communication, and Confidence. As Michael Bernoff teaches, it's like Einstein's formula, EMC2. If you practice and make an effort to strengthen each of those areas of your life, there's truly no stressor that can bring you down.

All of the challenges you are learning in this book will teach you how to upgrade your abilities and "level up" to meet and *exceed* the demands of daily life without crumbling under pressure. As my meditation teacher Emily Fletcher taught me, what you are learning is, "Adaptation Energy". We need ample self-care to support our minds and bodies to meet the challenges of our daily existence.

In addition to the stressors listed, there are environmental stressors most of us don't even consider that could be affecting our health as well. Are you unconsciously consuming heavy metals in your food? Are you unconsciously drinking medications, pesticides, dry-cleaner agents, and other toxins in your unfiltered tap water every day? (Gross, right?) Are you not breathing properly, causing the body to slouch and go into fight or flight, and/or breathing in junk air from a polluted environment? Even if you don't smoke, living in a big city can have a tremendously negative impact on your body's ability to get and maintain healthy immune function.

Maybe you are feeling anxious or depressed or angry all the time and can't quite put your finger on why. Your body's hormones, micronutrients, neurotransmitters, gut health and microbiome, immune function, liver health, and more all play a part in how you think, feel, and behave.

If you can't point to any particular outside driver of stress, it's so important to look at your labs with a qualified Functional Medicine provider and make sure you are giving your precious system what it needs. Deficiencies and poor internal functionality can lead to brain fog, fatigue, mood issues, depression, anxiety, and so many surface symptoms that we're unaware of unless it's deciphered in labs.

At the end of this book, you'll read my chapter "Wasting Precious Time" to understand the importance of not guessing and always testing to see what's going on internally. I know of patients Regan has helped get off antidepressants once they realize they are gluten intolerant, or correcting hormone dysregulation and being able to put on muscle, strengthen their libido, and reduce brain fog. Even people who didn't realize their anxiety, brain fog, and inflammatory issues were stemming from mold toxins in their home that, once eradicated, resolved their concerns. You'd be amazed what Functional Medicine can do for stress.

By the way, I can't *stress* this enough: if you aren't pooping at least once a day, and a healthy, comfortable bowel movement at that, constipation leads to stress on the body. Constipation not only feels very uncomfortable but can drive toxins back into your system when you need to be eliminating them. This is also why I always tell clients to include that in their daily Awareness journal. So many times, we "think" we are going regularly only to realize after the journal work that we are only going once every two to three days.

Step 2: Acknowledge

I've made the mistake of skipping this step when trying to solve issues/concerns in my own life. Skipping straight from Awareness to Action can lead me to feel impatient, angry, frustrated, a little desperate, and many times, this causes me to push down any emotions surrounding the initial concern.

To acknowledge something exists is not to admit defeat. Think of it as a spiritual practice of accepting what is before you seek to change it. Learning to be okay with where you are now and not living in past regret, nor future anxiety is one of the best things you can do. If you truly believed that support and answers were already on their way to the problem at hand, you'd feel immense relief instantly.

This is the perfect time to practice self-love, understanding, empathy, forgiveness, and laughter towards ourselves as human beings. Many times, our feelings about others are actually just a reflection of the turmoil in our inner world and what we feel and say to ourselves daily. If you were to check in with the thoughts going on in your head, you might find them to be a bit cruel and critical. That's okay; we've all experienced the inner critic.

Rather than adding emotion on top of emotion and feeling angry that you are angry or sad that you are sad, acknowledging reminds you that what you are experiencing is temporary, is "energy in motion", and that "this too shall pass". It's giving yourself a break for being human, zero guilt and shame. In doing this step, it becomes so much easier over time to take the next step from a place of calm, trust, and faith that you have what you need to move through and beyond whatever challenge you perceive.

Step 3: Action

Once you are aware of what is happening and acknowledge and give yourself some love, you are primed to take action from a much more gentle, kind, empowered place than had you skipped the second step and gone straight to "fixing yourself" or "manhandling the problem".

Use this strategy of the three As (Awareness, Acknowledgement, and Action) to move through any mental, emotional, communication, and confidence stressors you may experience and see what follows.

Now for Your First Challenge!

Every day for the next week (and beyond), establish a form of connection with another person in your life. It could be your spouse, a friend, family member, child, co-worker, anyone. Do one kind thing for someone each day that establishes a sense of connection. You could phone a friend and ask them to join you for game night, tell each other corny jokes (the more laughter, the better), surprise someone with a flower, a love note, or a note of gratitude.

All of these tips are meant to remind you to establish forms of positive connection each day in order to help stimulate vagal tone, feel positive emotions, and reduce the impact of stress that we've now learned.

Here's your first peptide idea to jump start your capabilities:

Peptides for Stress, Anxiety, and Emotional Food Dependency

Selank

This peptide has been used in place of anxiety meds. It's great for eating disorders, food addictions, and it can be used as a healthy self-soothing technique.

Selank is a branch of amino acids that work by expressing the gene for the GABA neurotransmitter.
www.frontiersin.org/articles/10.3389/fphar.2017.00089/full

In a study of 60 patients with anxiety, Selank was found to improve the emotional health of the participants and had positive impacts on their quality of life that lasted beyond the duration of the study.
pubmed.ncbi.nlm.nih.gov/25176261

Selank is administered as a nasal spray and is one of the best peptides that I've found for relieving that feeling of angst that can derail me from enjoying life. My wife has commented on the calm that she notices with it as well. I have some patients who use it as needed and others who wish to stay on it long term.

Another added benefit of using Selank is that it also carries anti-viral properties. One study showed that the replication of the influenza virus was stopped with the use of Selank. Its ability to equalize TH1/TH2/Treg cytokine pathways directly and indirectly through the central nervous system with no known side effects makes this a go-to with any concerns of viral infections, including COVID-19.

Chapter Three
Breathing

BREATHING

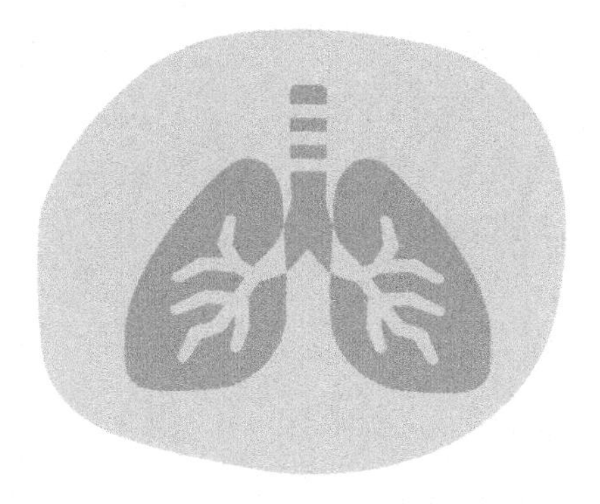

The Weight Loss Key You've Always Had

Mindset Number Three
I can breathe my way to my best health.

Sick Breath

Did you know mouth breathing can cause "sick breath" and a host of other problems within your body? Mouth breathing can weaken the diaphragm, a muscle that sits just below your ribcage.

Do an experiment right now to test your breath: breathe in as much air as you can through your nose and hold at the top. Now open your mouth and try to breathe in more air. If you can breathe in more, that means you're not breathing enough through your nose alone and are relying too much on "mouth breathing". Thank you, Dr. Dylan Knight, expert chiropractor, for this useful tool.

Another experiment is to tape your mouth shut while you sleep at night and see if it remains taped throughout the night. (No, we're not kidding!) If you wake up and have broken the tape, keep at it. This can help reduce snoring as well, so not only will it benefit *you* tremendously, but the quality of your partner's sleep as well.

The fastest way to die is to stop breathing.

Mouth breathing rots your teeth, doesn't allow for the oxygenation deep within your lungs, and makes your body more acidic.

Breathing correctly supports your body to expel waste products and can help reduce the likelihood of infections. While the nose is built as an internal filtration system to help eliminate toxins from entering the body, mouth breathing can increase infections, inflammation, and saturation of oxygen.

Nose breathing leads to increased nitric oxide production. Nitric oxide is a powerful tool to help increase parasympathetic tone, which we'll explain further next.

If that's not enough to convince you to switch to deep breaths through the nose, keep reading.

Parasympathetic Tone

Deep breathing can lower your blood pressure, reduce cortisol levels and increase parasympathetic tone. The parasympathetic tone is "rest and digest" mode. This helps burn fat, decrease inflammation, reduces issues within your nervous system, and reduces autoimmune flare-ups.

"Sympathetic mode" is your fight or flight response. We want to be in the parasympathetic mode most of the time and only in fight or flight response when we are truly in a dangerous situation that calls for it. ***Turning off your Sympathetic response and turning on your Parasympathetic response allows your body to heal.*** You already know how important this is, thanks to all that you learned in the chapter on "Stress".

Vagus & Phrenic Nerve Flow:

Another trip to Vagus! The vagus nerve runs from your brain on both sides of the body through every major organ down and up. If you always feel like you are in fight or flight mode and can't seem to relax, you might have sympathetic overstimulation from the vagus nerve energy not being able to move through. Strengthening your vagal tone through breath work allows you to get into "rest and digest" mode faster.

The Phrenic nerve runs from your neck down through your chest cavity into your heart and to the diaphragm. When the diaphragm gets less use, the nerve flow gets a lot more difficult.

Acidity vs. Alkalinity

Breathing through your nose also alkalizes your blood pH. With more acidic blood pH, your metabolism won't work as efficiently, you won't absorb the nutrients from food well with a diminished enzymatic response, and you'll have a harder time getting oxygen into your tissues, making your breath shallow (aka sick breathing).

When the blood becomes more alkaline, Calcium ions floating around in the blood go into hiding, binding onto large proteins in the blood called albumin. The body now experiences what it perceives to be a short-term low-calcium state, which causes increased firing in sensory and motor neurons.

The artificially low blood calcium now manifests in the neurological system as tingling sensations, smooth muscle contractions, and increased muscle tone. If you've ever not been able to move your mouth after a breathwork class, you know this feeling well! If you have done deep breathing before, or if while you are doing these exercises, you notice that tingling sensation, now you'll know why.

Anti-Inflammatory

Deep breathing also has an anti-inflammatory effect, while shallow breathing signals and increases inflammation in the body. A 2014 study out of Yale School of Medicine found that the epinephrine surge from deep breathing causes the innate immune system to increase its anti-inflammatory activity and dampen its proinflammatory activity. Subjects who were taught a breathwork routine had less severe inflammatory responses after exposure to IV bacterial toxins than those who didn't. The paper was the first in scientific literature to describe voluntary activation of the innate immune system. www.pnas.org/content/111/20/7379

A Note of Caution

The "high/loopy" feeling people experience during breathwork can be explained by hyperventilation and respiratory alkalosis. Increased blood pH decreases oxygen delivery to tissues; a phenomenon called the Bohr Effect. Within a minute of hyperventilation, the vessels in the brain constrict, reducing blood flow and oxygen delivery to the brain by 40%.

This is why it's important to **not** do these or other deep breathing techniques while driving, moving around, or in the shower, as it could make you lightheaded. Do them while seated comfortably or while lying down, and start slow.

Your Natural Energy Switch!

Who wouldn't love to "flip on their energy switch"?

Rather than depending on energy drinks, caffeine, sugar, and coffee, you can use oxygen to increase energy! When it comes to exercise and performance, when you feel heavy, and lactic acid builds up, you've gone from aerobic to anaerobic. Breathing properly and through your nose can lead to less lactic acid buildup and better recovery.

What's Your Air Quality?

Especially if you are in a polluted environment, experiencing forest fires, or living in a big city, it's important to have clean air to breathe in deep. We highly recommend checking out the EWG (Environmental Working Group) to look up product ratings for quality air filters for your home/work environment. You'll also learn more about what to look out for in the Chapter called "Love Your Liver".

How We Breathe

Breathing is the ultimate life source. Every day, we inhale and exhale on average 20,000 times to make sure we absorb sufficient oxygen. Oxygen (O_2) is delivered through our lungs, whereas carbon dioxide (CO_2) is just a byproduct (that your body nevertheless needs) and flows out.

Our lungs have a hierarchical branch structure that consists of two parts: the left and right lungs. The respiratory system supplies oxygen so that the air can be transported via the primary bronchus to the bronchiole (the smaller respiratory tract). These bronchioles effuse into lung bubbles, where oxygen and blood cohere. During this diffusion, O_2 is absorbed via the blood, whereas CO_2 is dissolved. This process is a biological process known as gas exchange. After this exchange, oxygen-rich blood is transported to enter the body cells.

If your CO_2 levels are elevated, we know you are a mouth breather! This is yet another reason it's important to run labs and have them read by a provider.

Breathing for Immunity

Now more than ever, it's so important to activate the immune system. Your Thymus gland is a part of this system, creating Lymphocytes (white blood cells) that protect the body from infections. However, the thymus gland shrinks as you age, so it's important to care for it! You can activate it with a simple routine.

To locate it, draw a line with your finger between your nipples and land in the center of your sternum. Move your finger a couple of inches up towards your neck. Start lightly tapping on this area. Make sure as you tap that you inhale twice as long as you exhale. Tap and breathe, and you are activating your thymus gland.

Breathing to Relax

Breathing is one of the best ways to turn down the sympathetic nervous system response and activate parasympathetic tone.

In *Zen Bow, Zen Arrow* by John Stevens, a teacher of archery shows his students an exercise of breathing to open up the ribcage, exhale, and how much more easily it allows him to shoot his arrow. The only way to hit your target is to breathe properly!

We also highly recommend the book called *Breath: The New Science of a Lost Art* by James Nestor, which goes into even more detail about the incredible benefits of breathing.

Breathing Will Change Your Posture

Most people slouch. Do a little experiment and try to breathe deep from a slouched position. Does it feel strange? Does it make it harder? It just doesn't work.

Now stand up for a moment, and put your pinkies on your hip bones and your thumbs on your ribcage. Now inhale through your nose and lift your ribcage up as you breathe. Keep your head and neck straight, as if there is a fishing line at the top center of your head, pulling you gently upward.

Now, to help you feel less hunched over, try this. Put your arms out in front of you, rounded, as if you are holding a big beach ball. Then pull your arms down and back on either side of your torso, with your fists up and sliding against your ribcage. You should feel your shoulder blades pull down and back at the same time. Make that motion on the inhale through your nose, and do your "beach ball arms," rounding your spine on the exhale breath. This will help loosen and strengthen the trapezius muscles that support your posture. Weak, tight trapezius muscles combined with tight, tense shoulders, create the perfect storm for a rounded, hunched posture. This will help open you up.

Given our society's tendency to sit most of the day, whether it's in a car, during our commute, or at a computer desk, this further increases the hunched posture. We crane our neck towards the computer, we tighten our hip flexors sitting all day, and weaken our buttocks. We tense and tighten as we go into sympathetic mode when a car cuts in front of us or we receive an email that triggers us. We crane our necks looking down at our smartphones, and put the phone against our shoulder up to our ear while we use our hands to balance multiple things. We may sit on the couch in a slouched position while we watch television.

It's really important to be aware of posture as much as possible and to remind ourselves and teach ourselves how to keep aligned posture no matter what the activity. Also, taking breaks to stand up, stretch, and walk at least once an hour is so important for our functional movement.

If you would love to learn more about how to keep alignment and optimal posture no matter what activity you are doing, we highly recommend working with a physical therapist and chiropractor. While we offer both, if we aren't in your area, you can check what is near you with a Google search, check-in with us as we may have referrals, or try Alexander Technique! It's meant to help you move through life's activities in a more relaxed and comfortable way, as nature intended.

When I was having back and neck issues after doing a Broadway National Tour, a combination of physical therapy, deep tissue massage, and Alexander Technique rocked my world and eliminated the pain. The exercises to loosen and strengthen certain muscle groups that had grown tense or weak were so helpful. I had no idea that my shoulders were rounded partially because my front pectoral muscles were so tight, and the trapezius muscles weakened and tight. Combined, it was pulling my shoulders forward, causing discomfort.

When learning Alexander Technique, they will have you stand as you normally would comfortably and look in the mirror. I noticed immediately that, while the position was comfortable, my posture was not at all ideal. When standing with correct postural alignment, looking in the mirror, I could see the difference, but it felt uncomfortable as if I were straining. Certain muscle groups had grown comfortable in the incorrect position and uncomfortable when correctly aligned.

Breathing for Mental and Emotional Health

In *Peace Is Every Step* by Thich Nhat Hanh, he mentioned the great importance of breath, bringing you back to present moment awareness, away from regrets of the past or fears of the future.

The best part of conscious breathing is that it can be done any time, from anywhere! Are you sitting in traffic and getting irritated, wishing you could teleport home? Focus on some deep belly diaphragmatic breathing. Eating any meal is the perfect time to consciously breathe and savor each bite. Do you notice you are drifting in thought when you are speaking to a friend rather than listening? Come back to the breath and focus on being present, and you're well on your way to far better communication and connection.

If this creates a powerful "why statement" for you, Thich Nhat Hanh recommends a deep breath in order to restore calm, peace, joy, and love to your state of being. We are always chasing after these states of being, yet we tend to approach it by chasing after things outside of our being. You can be happy, content, and at peace at any time, simply by returning to your breath.

Have you ever approached a conflict in relation to others and reacted quickly to a trigger, regretting what you said or did after the fact? What's a great way to prevent that in the future? Stop *before* you react, sit comfortably or even walk if that's best, and do ten deep breaths. If you're still feeling a bit worked up, do it once more. It's guaranteed you will re-approach the situation or conversation from a much calmer place, triggering the best of yourself.

Breathing in a shallow way can actually send a signal to the body to go into fight or flight, even if nothing dangerous is happening. By training the body to breathe properly, we set the stage for the body to believe it's safe, and the mind follows suit as well.

Breathing for Asthma

When your lungs go into spasm, it's a very uncomfortable feeling.

Part of what these exercises do is to retrain your lungs on how to behave. Once you start getting the proper O_2 and CO_2 exchange, the alveoli (tiny air sacs of the lungs) have fewer mucosal secretions and less phlegm which can cause spasms. When you take a deep breath, your diaphragm is contracting. Getting it to contract and strengthen will alleviate a lot of asthma.

This can absolutely help alleviate and relieve asthmatic stress, especially during exercise.

Breathing for Incontinence

This entire experience will strengthen your diaphragm. When you think of your core, what do you think of?

When asked this question, most will respond with the muscles in your torso and back. Have you ever thought of it from a 3-D perspective, like a can? Your core is composed of a "top" (your diaphragm) and a "bottom" (your pelvic floor). This is something Dr. Dylan Knight taught us, one of our expert chiropractors.

After childbirth and over time, many women may experience incontinence, which is loss of bladder control. While pelvic floor exercises like Kegels are very supportive of the pelvic floor, the top (diaphragm muscle) tends to be ignored.

Do you ever bend down and feel like your hip catches? You feel strain and pressure on the "outside" parts of the can.

If you are struggling with incontinence and pelvic floor exercises alone aren't producing the results you are looking for, start strengthening your diaphragm with breath work! Dylan has seen this work for his clients struggling with incontinence by approaching core strength from all angles. You can retrain your muscles with the repetition of proper breathing.

Breathing and Pain

The diaphragm is your main respiratory muscle. Not utilizing your diaphragm properly makes other muscle groups kick in as your secondary or emergency respiratory group and makes it even harder to breathe properly. It's your "back-up" system, and it's not meant to take the lead.

Take a moment. Do you feel tightness between your collar bones up to your trap muscle? If your neck is chronically tight, one of the things that could be happening is poor respiration. Your head tilts forward, and this can increase headaches and neck pain. When your head comes forward, the body starts to work harder.

The nervous system is an electrical system. Think of it, quite literally, as a conduction unit. If the wires leading to the light bulb aren't properly set up to allow for the energy to move, the light won't shine. Your body, when properly aligned, is an energy-producing machine. You can relax it and retrain your body with proper diaphragmatic breathing.

Try this exercise. Put your dominant hand on your belly and your opposite hand on your chest. You can be seated or lying down. As you breathe in through your nose, taking a deep belly breath, push with your dominant hand against your belly as the air fills up. Then purse your lips and breath out at the top. Repeat this just five times. Now, go back to your collar bone and revisit the same trap muscles you did before. Do you notice less tightness? That's the power of your breath.

How did that happen? You were activating your primary respiratory system with diaphragmatic breathing, rather than the overuse of your secondary system that led to the tight muscle groups to begin with.

Breathing for Osteoporosis

Are you struggling with Osteoporosis/Osteopenia, or know of someone who has been diagnosed? If you don't activate calcium and phosphorus, then taking more as a supplement can be futile, as you aren't properly absorbing it. Alkalizing your blood helps calcium get into the muscle and into your bones, helping you become stronger.

Regan's breath work allows him to athletically perform at his best and to handle his cold plunges with strength and ease (more on that later).

Breathing and Sleep

Using these breathing exercises can reduce sleep apnea, snoring, and poor-quality sleep.

Diminished sleep quality leads to a host of issues, including impaired cognition, higher levels of anxiety, increased stroke risk, increased risk for diabetes, increased symptoms of depression, weight gain, and increased risk for heart disease and breast cancer. If you sleep six hours or less a night, your risk of stroke increases four times!

Recent studies have shown snoring in children is significantly associated with poor academic performance, hyperactivity, as well as daytime sleepiness. www.ncbi.nlm.nih.gov/pmc/articles/PMC5753659

Breathing and Brain Detox

Believe it or not, your brain is actually more active while you sleep than it is by day!

Your brain uses 20% of electrical energy while you are awake vs. 25% while you are sleeping. This metabolic activity requires constant cleansing, which mostly takes place while you sleep.

The brain's natural "garbage disposal" is found in the cerebrospinal fluid (CSF), a naturally occurring fluid the brain uses to "wash off" biological waste products, which then gets dumped into general circulation. This internal plumbing system is called the glymphatic system.

When you have sleep apnea or snore, you lose the ability to remove excess waste from the brain, which can build up amyloid plaques and inflammation. Not only proper breathing but proper positioning while sleeping has a huge impact on this detox process. Research tells us that people with neurodegenerative conditions spend almost twice as much time on their backs while sleeping.

Studies have shown the influence of body posture on the brain-wide transport of inert tracers of anesthetized rodents. The major finding of the study was that waste, including Aβ removal, was most efficient in the lateral position (sleeping on your side) compared with the prone position (sleeping on your back). The glymphatic system is most effective in the lateral position, as was confirmed in MRIs. (*J. Neurosci.* 2015 AUG. 5)

Suggestions

- Do the exercises taught above.
- Sleep on your side and not on your back.
- Get hypoallergenic pillows and clean them often. You can put them in the sun to kill off growths of bacteria/mold.
- Get air filters for your home/work environments.
- You can get charcoal sticks to absorb odors.
- Fill your home and work environment with plants! That, too, cleanses your air naturally.

- Don't toxify your own air with fragrances, chemicals, perfumes, allergens, dust, burning scented candles, etc.
- Practice great posture, and get assistance from professionals if you are having difficulty

Are you ready? Are you convinced of the importance of breathing for optimal function?

Wim Hof is a man who is intrinsically linked with the words cold, breathing, and immune system. In the past few years, he has become famous for being able to withstand sub-zero temperatures without protection from the elements, climbing Mt Everest in shorts! The "Iceman" has proven how he can change his body in ways previously considered to be out of our control.

Challenge 2: Try diaphragmatic breath work for 2.5 to five minutes. Lie on your back with your legs propped up by a pillow. Put one hand on your belly, one on your chest. Breath in through the nose slowly, out through the mouth. Try pushing the hand against your belly as you inhale through the nose to make your diaphragm work!

Then do Wim Hof's breathing exercise in the morning and at night. Each round (three rounds making up one breathing exercise) is thirty breaths in and out. Breath in through your nose and out through pursed lips. On the thirtieth exhale, let all the air out and hold without breathing in. Aim for a 60-second hold to start. If you need to breathe in before you hit 60 seconds on a timer, please do! You can work your way up to 60 seconds and beyond.

Once you breathe in, hold at the top of the breath for 15 seconds, then slowly let the air out and come back to the start. Repeat two more times, and then lie comfortably and bring your attention back to slow, steady breathing. I highly recommend doing this with Wim's guided video on YouTube here: www.youtube.com/watch?v=tybOi4hjZFQ

This releases a chemical called DMT, triggering a euphoric feeling. This is similar to the effects of psychedelics. Oxytocin (loving feeling) also gets released.

If you need a guided tutorial, Wim Hof has great free videos on YouTube and an application you can download and trial. It allows you to track your progress with breath work as well as his other suggested tools like meditation, push-ups and stretching.

As mentioned, do not do this while driving, moving, or in the shower. Do this either seated or while lying on your back. You might feel that tingling sensation in your hands and feet, and that is normal!

Make note of the positive changes you notice as the challenge goes. Write down your wins and feel the rewards from your effort.

Peptides for Lung Capacity, Immune Function, and Longevity

You have an immune treasure next to your lungs called the thymus gland. Every time you breathe, you stimulate blood flow for immune cell production. This gland trains your white blood cells, specifically, your T-lymphocytes, which are key defense cells for viral and other types of infection, to recognize threats. The thymus gland works through peptide pathways like thymosin alpha-1, Thymulin, Thymosin beta-4, or the actin-binding potential-7 (APB-7) pathway.

As we age, our thymus gland shrinks, which can leave our immune system with less intelligent capability to recognize and combat infections.
www.endocrineweb.com/endocrinology/overview-thymus

That's why using peptides like Thymulin-Zinc, Thymosin Alpha 1, or ABP-7 during times of immune stress can be helpful in training each of your new white blood cells in their duties of recognizing the threat and responding in a natural way. Researchers have found ways to bypass aging with the use of peptides that modulate enhanced immune intelligence.
www.sciencedirect.com/science/article/abs/pii/089684119290152G

Chapter Four
Sugar

If You Do Nothing Else, Do This One Thing

Mindset Number Four
I make informed choices about everything I consume. I put my future health first rather than momentary satisfaction.

Oh, sugar. By now, you should be a five-letter swear word.

Growing up, I was no stranger to sugar in its many forms: boxed and bagged products, pop (I'm from Ohio, and we say "pop", not "soda".), desserts, candies, and more.

I'll never forget my days in college when I believed it was okay to use Splenda (that it was way better for my health) and all sorts of fake sweeteners to scratch the itch I had for sweets. I'd eventually cave and have the real stuff on the weekends, at parties, and at holiday gatherings.

Cutting it out entirely seemed impossible to me then. I would tell myself I wouldn't eat it at gatherings using sheer willpower or when going home for a holiday: "Not this time!" Sure enough, the addictive behavioral pattern would kick in, and I'd be pounding my favorite cookies, chocolate, desserts, and snacks. That vicious cycle would leave me feeling deep guilt and shame, and I'd "get back on track" by putting myself on a low-calorie, low-fat diet with fake sweeteners and an intense workout routine.

I also began binge eating until I felt painfully full in private. I had black-and-white thinking around dieting and a poor relationship with my body and food. It was a major struggle in my life from around ages 18 to 24 and one that not many knew about. I hid it well with a petite frame and being very active, to the point where even my therapist didn't believe me when I admitted my problem.

I would read books about binge eating to try and glean what I needed to make the change for the better, for good, but nothing worked. I remember a time when I thought to myself, "Maybe this is just something I'll need to manage and live with for the rest of my life." That thought was painful, and I'm glad I refused to accept it.

Fast forward to the late fall of 2014 in New York City. I had graduated from my health coaching program and was working with clients and a business coach. Despite all the many healthy changes I had made during my schooling, though, I was still stressed out, burnt out, and turned to food for comfort.

My business coach invited me to attend a free meditation class. I thought, "Well, why not?" I love health and wellness, and while the Deepak Chopra and Oprah 21-day meditation challenges had not had a profound effect on me, I was curious.

That night, I listened as Emily Fletcher, a previous Broadway performer, shared her journey about becoming a meditation teacher after learning the practice changed her life. It almost seemed too good to be true, but I knew I had a lot of stress built up over many years that needed undoing, and I needed something powerful to help me accomplish that. I liked that this didn't seek to fight the stress consciously but rather sit and let the conscious chatter quiet for a while.

That weekend, I learned to meditate. Emily told our class to expect there to be some "side effects" of unstressing. Some tears or emotions that had been built up inside might finally have a chance to come out. That's okay. You might feel tired and need some extra naps as you get started (this was true for me). That's okay too. I liked how gentle it was and that the only goal of being a meditator was not to be a good meditator but rather to do it in order to get better at life. No smartphone, loud beeping timers, or guided voice in my ear was needed. I've since meditated under trees, on trains, and even in a tiny supply closet that I squeezed myself into for privacy at one of my old jobs.

About six months after starting meditation, I was in the midst of a new job. Was I still stressed out? Absolutely. The stress never vanished, but it hit me one day: "Oh my. I haven't binged food since I started meditating." That was a moment I'll never forget. The problem (whatever it was) had vanished. Would I still crave sugar at times and indulge or overeat a little on occasion? Yes, but I was able to stop myself before the guilt, shame, and anxiety that drove me to eat in excess as if my belly was a bottomless pit set in. The bingeing was completely gone.

I also noticed, within my first year of being a meditator, that I was no longer experiencing motion sickness on planes. Certain flights would give me such nausea and vertigo for 24 hours afterward that I'd take a baby dose of Dramamine to prevent it. Do you know what that did? Nothing but make me want to pass out for 24 hours. Either way, I felt awful. Meditating on takeoff and landing, I no longer felt ill.

Now, seven years later, still meditating, I still don't experience binge-eating episodes or motion sickness on planes. Did meditation solve all of my problems? Not at all, but it gave me the ability to separate myself from my emotions just long enough to take a glance at them. I no longer feel as triggered by things that used to upset me. I felt a bit more chill. That, coupled with the above benefits, made it worth the time.

For other classmates of mine, meditation helped them with a variety of concerns, including insomnia, headaches, irregular periods/painful cramps, anxiety, depression, and a lot more. If I were to guess how it managed to get me less addicted to food, I'd say it was the stress component. Unwinding allowed me to relax more and allowed my body to follow suit.

If you struggle with an eating disorder, while meditation may not be the end-all-be-all solution for you, it's 100% recommended on your healing journey. That, along with emotional freedom tapping, yoga, speaking with a qualified therapist who specializes in supporting people with eating disorders, learning self-care techniques, and private support groups like Overeaters Anonymous, are all available today. That first step towards healing begins when you open yourself up to receiving help and learning some self-care as well.

I share this story in case you find, as you are reading this that the idea of letting go of your favorite junk foods, sugary foods, or routines feels triggering. I have felt the same way. Any time in the past I was encouraged to let go of something in order to see how I'd feel without it (but I loved it), I'd resist that change like hell. That is until I had suffered long enough that the change was a welcome relief to the self-sabotage of continuing to do the same thing, expecting different results. It's funny how, for many, it takes being sick of feeling sick to get us to change our ways.

While food is meant to be nourishing, savored, and enjoyed with those you love, it's not meant to cause you internal distress, mentally or physically. If you are clinging to something you know doesn't serve you, ask yourself, "Where will I be one year from now if nothing changes? What would life be like if I weren't addicted to food? How might I enjoy parties and not feel anxious about temptations? How might I enjoy life more if I had a healthy relationship with food?"

Now, let's dive into the knowledge you need to see how impactful this one habit alone will be in your life.

On average, 63% of calories consumed in the U.S. are from processed foods.

Did you also know that the same percentage of Americans are overweight? That number is way too high, and the sad part is we all know it's preventable.

What do sugar, junk foods, and artificial sweeteners do to the body?

It can create brain fog, fatigue from the blood sugar highs and lows, blood sugar irregularities that can lead to diabetes, heart conditions, weight gain, cancer, and other diseases. Blood sugar issues can also lead to mood swings, poor immune system function leading to a higher likelihood of getting sick, exhaustion, and further addiction and dependency on these very ingredients, causing a vicious cycle. It was no surprise that sugar is as addicting, if not more so than cocaine.
pubmed.ncbi.nlm.nih.gov/

Have you ever taken a short break from sugar only to go back and realize that things you had previously eaten now taste grossly sweet? That's because your taste buds can and do change with time, depending on what you are eating. Just like you can become so adjusted to alcohol that you need more to feel a buzz, you can also adjust to the point where your body rejects these things in excess. You eventually start to crave food the way nature intended.

Did you know that there are more than 50 different names for sugar? That doesn't even include artificial sweeteners. Check out the list below. Learning what your food labels are actually telling you is one of the best things you can do for your health so that you aren't blindly buying and eating sugar-laden foods.

56 NAMES FOR SUGAR

Blackstrap Molasses

Cane Sugar

Confectioner's Sugar

Date Sugar

Diastatic Malt

Florida Crystals

Galactos

Golden Syrup

Icing Sugar

Maltodextrin

Muscovado

Refiner's Syrup Sugar

Barbados Sugar

Agave Nectar

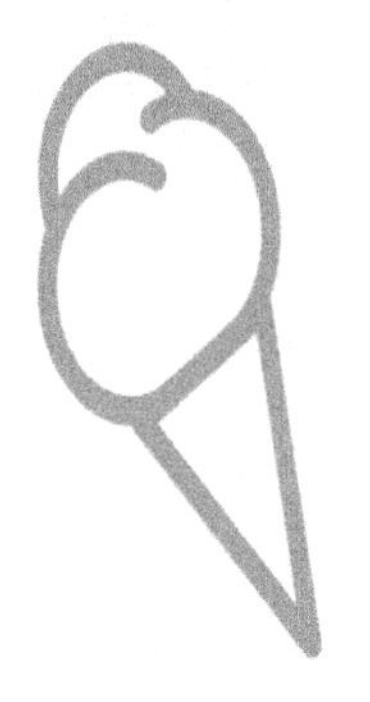

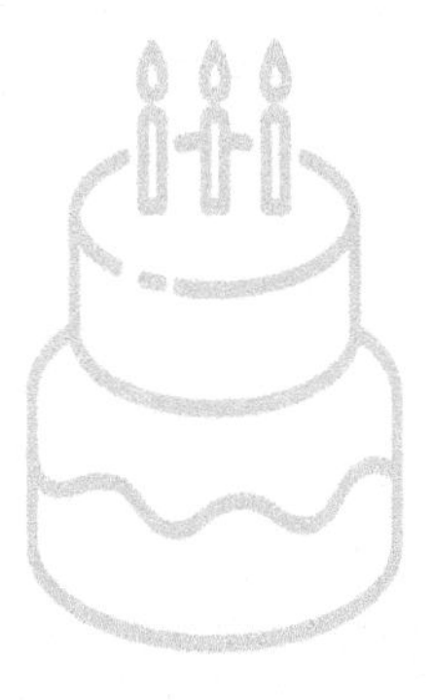

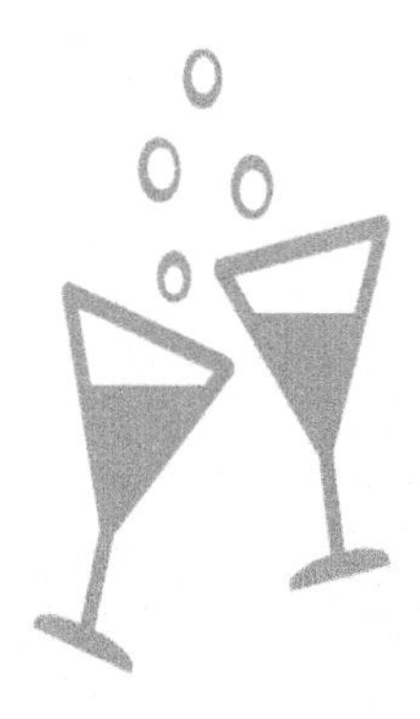

Organic Raw Sugar

Rice Syrup

Treacle

Barley Malt

Buttered Syrup

Carob Syrup

Corn Syrup Solids

Dextran

Ethyl Maltol

Fruit Juice

Glucose Solids

Lactose

Maple Syrup

Maltose

56 NAMES FOR SUGAR

Beet Sugar

Cane Juice Crystals

Castor Sugar

Crystalline Fructose

Dextrose

Evaporated Cane Juice

Golden Sugar

Malt Syrup

Caramel

Corn Syrup

High Fructose Corn Syrup

Demerara Sugar

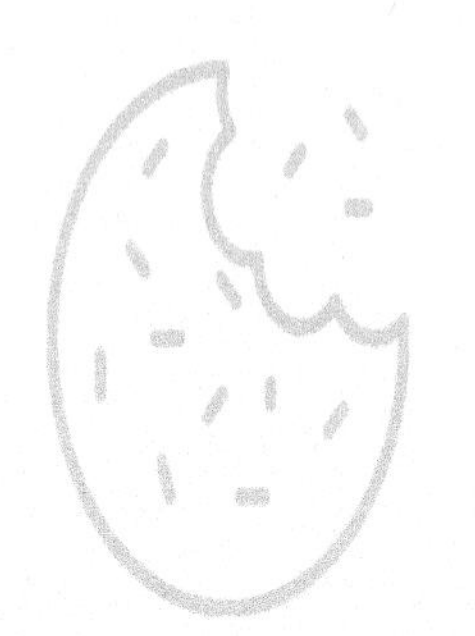

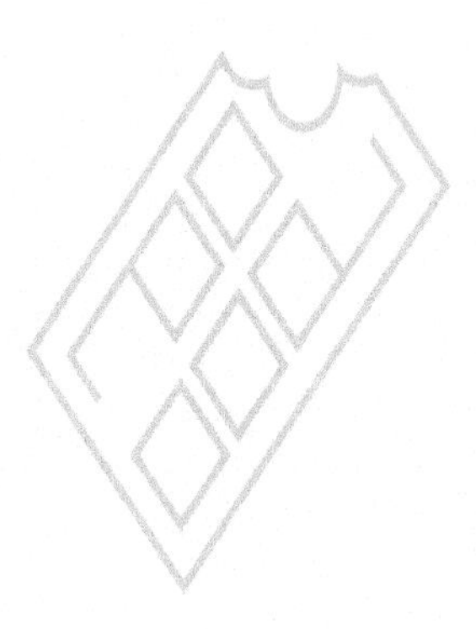

Sorghum Syrup

Diatase

Fructose

Grape Sugar

Invert Sugar

Molasses

Raw Sugar

Sucrose

Honey

Yellow Sugar

Brown Sugar

Turbinado Sugar

Panocha

Between the laundry list of names for sugar alone, not to mention the other chemicals and artificial sweeteners we want you to be aware of, it can easily get overwhelming.

That's why we love to use one of the best resources for sourcing safe things to eat and drink called the Environmental Working Group, www.ewg.org. They also have a great app you can use on the go. They provide a rating for food, beverages, and home products to help you make informed choices. You don't have to memorize all the many chemicals and ingredients to avoid.

MSG "Monosodium Glutamate" is another ingredient in foods to watch out for. We wanted you to be aware of its many names well. MSG is a flavor enhancer that is considered "GRAS" (Generally Recognized As Safe) by the FDA but can cause weight gain as it makes you want to eat more. It tends to show up in processed junk foods.

HIDDEN NAMES FOR MSG

MONOSODIUM GLUTAMATE

GELATIN

YEAST FOOD OR NUTRIENT

SODIUM CASEINATE

YEAST FOOD OR NUTRIENT

CALCIUM CASEINATE

AUTOLYZED PLANT PROTEIN

HYDROLYZED VEGETABLE PROTEIN (HVP)

GLUTAMATE

TEXTURED PROTEIN

AUTOLYZED YEAST

HYDROLYZED PLANT PROTEIN (HPP)

YEAST EXTRACT

MONOPOTASSIUM GLUTAMATE

Artificial sweeteners are just as detrimental and have many different names. Aim for monk fruit or organic stevia (nothing else added) to help with getting off sugar.

- Aspartame (Equal, NutraSweet). It's mostly used to sweeten diet soft drinks.
- Saccharin (Sweet 'N Low, Sugar Twin). It's used in many diet foods and drinks.
- Sucralose (Splenda). It's in many diet foods and drinks.
- Acesulfame K (Sunett). It's often combined with saccharin in diet soft drinks.
- Stevia with other ingredients in brands like Truvia.

Junk Food

More than 95% of chronic diseases are caused by food choices, toxic food ingredients, nutritional deficiencies, and lack of physical exercise.

Be very careful when reading labels, as they tend to be misleading in their advertising to get you to buy the product. It's frustrating when you learn how many food products are allowed to advertise with false claims. The average shopper believes a food product is healthy if it says "natural" or has other earthly terms on the label when in actuality, it is not.

Since the majority of people aren't provided in-depth knowledge of nutrition, nor do people have the time to memorize all the names of ingredients and their meanings, many are left believing what the box or bag has to say on the surface.

Here are some top terms you will most likely come across at the grocery store, what each means, and what to truly lookout for a while shopping:

*Indicates information extracted from this *Healthline* article by Adda Bjarnadottir, MS, RDN (Ice), Updated on August 19, 2020.

- **Gluten-free:** while seeing the "certified gluten-free" label brings relief to someone with celiac disease who must avoid it at all cost, this does not signify "healthy". Many boxed and bagged products nowadays are made gluten-free for those diagnosed with celiac disease, gluten intolerance, or gluten sensitivity.

  I love that there are options, but all it really means is that the protein "gluten" found in many foods (not just grains) is not in the product. That's not an indicator that it's now healthy. Say you have gluten-free cookies, but it has a long list of other ingredients and preservatives you've never seen before, sugar or artificial sweeteners added, and maybe other non-gluten-containing foods like processed corn, soy, white rice flour, etc. You have a recipe for a very unhealthy food being marketed as a solid option.

- **Natural:** *This does not necessarily mean that the product resembles anything natural. It simply indicates that, at one point, the manufacturer worked with a natural source like apples or rice.

- **Organic:** While we now have certification requirements that must be followed in order for a company to use the certified organic green label, this too doesn't tell us if it's healthy. This is best used for the "dirty dozen" foods as shared by the EWG. However, any food can follow organic requirements and still be filled with sugar, gluten, and other pro-inflammatory foods by nature.
- **Whole Grain:** Why would a product be listed as "Whole grain" in the first place? In many processed products, like cereals, for example, the grain that is used is pulverized and has the outer fibrous part removed, making it no longer the whole food it once was. What you are left with is the part of the grain that can quickly be broken down by the body, easily spiking your blood sugar, and has a lot of the original nutritional value removed.

  Have you noticed that it will also say on cereal boxes "Enriched" in the ingredients label? That's because they've added nutrients back into the product after processing (i.e., you'll notice vitamins and minerals listed on boxed cereals). Bleached products are treated with chemicals to speed up aging, whereas unbleached are not. How lovely. Cereal is probably one of the worst perpetrators of misleading language in advertising, considering it usually contains some form of sugar, chemicals, additives, gluten, dyes, and more. Not only is this dangerous for your health but for the majority of children to whom these products are marketed to. Remember, chemicals and additives that are GRAS might be studied for safely on their own, but not taking into account the chemicals on top of chemicals you could be consuming in one meal, like a bowl of cereal.

- **Sugar-Free/No Sugar Added:** Sugar-free may mean that an artificial sweetener was added, which isn't considered sugar. No sugar added doesn't mean there is no sugar, but rather that they haven't added sugar on top of what is either naturally occurring in the product or the artificial sweeteners that aren't regular sugar by definition.

  You might need to read that twice; that's how confusing it is. Be on the lookout for sugar or artificial sweeteners snuck into these and many other products that you may not expect: salad dressings, yogurts, nut milk, regular milk, crackers, breads, bacon (yes, bacon and other meats may have sugar added), oatmeal, kombucha tends to have a lot of added sugar and doesn't need it, juice drinks (It might say no sugar added, but juicing fruits and/or doing full fruit smoothies is a LOT of sugar in a sitting.), snack foods, protein bars (a big one for sugar), protein powders, etc.

- **Original/Plain/Unflavored:** Equally confusing, this doesn't mean the product doesn't have sugar. Just that it's meant to be plain in taste without a flavor like strawberry, chocolate, and vanilla. If you want no sugar, you have to look for "Unsweetened" on the label.

- **Sugar Alcohol:** Confusing name, as it's not actual sugar! This is a sugar substitute that provides a lot of sweetness.

  Examples: Xylitol, Erythritol, Sorbitol, Mannitol, etc. If eating foods that contain sugar alcohol gives you stomach upset, pull it out.

- **Keto:** Keto is a type of diet that is comprised of mostly healthy fat, only about 10 to 15% protein, and very little carbohydrates from low-carb vegetables like leafy greens. Your body is meant to go into "ketosis," where it starts to burn fat for fuel rather than sugar. Processed Keto foods can still have certain preservatives, additives, and sweeteners added, but it does tend to be better than most junk foods.

- **Paleo:** This is another type of diet that cuts out foods that weren't in alignment with the Paleolithic Era. Think cavemen eating meat, berries, vegetables, and fats rather than post-industrialized foods containing grain, legumes, and other processed foods. While this, like Keto, can be done properly, don't just assume because it's Paleo that it is healthy. These foods can still contain a lot of sugar from sources like honey, maple syrup, etc. The best you can do with either diet is to eat clean, whole foods without added sugar.

- **Whole 30 Approved:** Whole 30 is a diet that requires eating only whole food ingredients for a minimum of 30 days, not including things like grain, legumes, sugar, alcohol, and especially no chemicals or additives. It is similar to paleo and helps get away from all bagged, boxed, and bottled processed food and drink products. Just pay close attention as fruits high in sugar and things like dates may still be approved but are not meant to be overeaten.

- **DRI:** Daily Recommended Intake of any micronutrient or macronutrient is very generic and not very informative. It doesn't take into account gender, body size, where your micronutrient levels currently are, or the fact that your body also must absorb the nutrients properly in order to get the benefits. It's best to get your blood work done, know what you are truly deficient in, and bring it up to optimal levels with the guidance of a functional medicine provider.
- **Vegan:** This diet avoids all meat products as well as dairy, eggs, fish, and in some cases, even honey. Some vegetarians may still partake in eggs (ovo-vegetarians), fish (pescatarians), dairy (lacto-vegetarians), and/or honey. Just remember, things like wheat, corn, soy, and sugar are all technically vegan because they don't come from animal products. If you see a vegan dessert, that means it's free of butter and eggs. That doesn't mean it's free of inflammatory vegetables oils, high fructose corn syrup, table sugar, or preservatives, additives, etc.
- **Non-GMO (Non-Genetically Modified Foods):** Yes, that means that many foods nowadays are genetically modified in a lab. While this hasn't been officially proven to be detrimental to people's health, the non-GMO project seeks to keep the

public informed of what they are eating so that we all can make the choice of whether we want "franken-food" or not. You can learn more about them and about GMOs here: www.nongmoproject.org

- **Trans Fat:** Artificially processed fats that, unlike so many food additives, chemicals, and ingredients, have been deemed unhealthy for human consumption and removed from products as a result. You may see "No trans fat" on certain labels. It also has to be listed on products so you can check and see what your nutrition facts tell you of the trans fat within the product. If it has any for any reason, be sure to avoid it.
- **Preservatives:** While these give food items a longer shelf life, food is meant to mold and break down. It's like the McDonald's experiment. An organic grass-fed burger, when left out, will mold and break down quickly. A McDonald's burger and fries will look pretty much the same for weeks. That's not natural! You can keep things frozen to preserve them longer or seek to buy only what you need so as not to end up with rotten food waste.
- **Antibiotics and Growth Hormones:** If you weren't already informed of this, this is crucial. Stop buying factory-farmed meats, fish, and dairy immediately. There are plenty of documentaries available now to show you what's really going on in these farming environments, including the injection of growth hormones into animals to get them bigger before slaughter and the use of antibiotics when sick. They

are kept in awful environments and not allowed to roam freely. They are fed grains to fatten them up. What they consume, you consume when you eat them. Not to mention fish that are kept in small dirty, crowded water environments and later injected to make them look more healthy in color, like salmon, before it gets to the store. I will go much more in-depth on this in the chapter on Protein.

While the focus thus far has been on what to avoid, there are SO many clean whole foods we highly recommend eating! Experiment with and explore the outer edges of your grocery store.

All the colors of the rainbow in the produce section, different organic meats with no growth hormones or antibiotics added, wild-caught fish, healthy fats from dry roasted/raw nuts, seeds, avocados, unprocessed oils, etc. are all fantastic options. Eating in season is also great as it's the way nature intended for us to eat certain foods and get certain nutrients depending on where we live and the time of year. You can get local fresh seasonal produce from your farmer's market, a CSA, and/or look up a list of what foods are in peak season, depending on the time of year.

You can also begin to swap those junk foods above or ones you are used to with some better whole-food snacks, including on-the-go travel options:

- Epic protein bars
- Lily's dark chocolate (stevia sweetened)

- Lakanto Monk Fruit products
- Organic coffee
- Simple Mills crackers or Pizza Dough
- Peak Performance bars: No sweeteners added at all, and great carb, protein, fat, and fiber ratio!
- Primal Kitchen dressings and collagen bars: Still make sure no sugar is added
- Unsweetened nut milks without preservatives like 3 Trees, Joi, or you can actually make some with a blender and save a lot of money on those bottled/boxed products!
- Check out some homemade bars/snacks that also save a lot of money, like Elana's Pantry or Essence of Jessie!

Why are organic products more expensive than cheap foods that are bad for you?

The government subsidizes crops that make up a lot of processed foods on the market, like wheat, corn, sugar, and soy. They are laden with pesticides, and when ground up, remove a lot of the natural fiber in the whole food that would slow things down. Suddenly, these wheat, corn, and soy-based products are blood sugar spiking machines.

Take boxed cereals, for example. The majority of these are made with those three ingredients and/or rice plus added sugar, colored dyes, and then "enriched" with vitamins and minerals. They're super cheap to make and made to fly off the shelves.

How is this legal?

Many chemicals are GRAS (generally recognized as safe) but aren't tested in combination with others. We're not just consuming single chemicals in tiny doses. We're accumulating chemicals quickly via all the many chemicals in our food, drinks, tap water, makeup products, body products, household cleaners, and more.

This can lead to what's called xenoestrogen buildup. Chemicals that mimic estrogen in the body can confuse the body into producing less of its own or accumulate too high of levels than the body can manage.

Suggestions:

- Follow Michael Pollen's Food Rules: Eat real food (whole food ingredients that you can recognize, five or fewer on a food label), not too much, and mostly plants.
- Swaps sugars for organic stevia or monk fruit.
- Read your labels and use the guidance above.
- Avoid the inner aisles of the grocery store and stick to the produce, meat/poultry section, eggs, and items that don't even have much of a label
- Pick out delicious recipes and make your grocery list in advance. Meal prep will save you time and money and help you avoid temptation and crashes where you feel starved!
- Use the EWG app on the go-to vet products.

- Slowly but surely, start to swap any cleaning, body, or makeup products you have that don't have safe EWG ratings with products that do! One at a time, you'll eventually get everything in alignment.
- We talk more about chemicals to be aware of in your environment in the "Love Your Liver" chapter and what to do about it.

Challenge: No junk food, sugar, artificial sweeteners, or foods with added chemicals in the ingredients list.

If you are a bit addicted/very used to certain products with fake/regular sugars, start with simply cleaning out your kitchen. Make this easier on yourself by removing temptation from your immediate environment. Don't add anything at the grocery store on this list, either. Out of sight, out of mind.

Make a list of what you plan to get at the grocery store before you go, sticking to whole foods, and avoid the aisles where you know your favorite snacks, desserts, and treats are located. If you need to order your groceries for delivery, that works too! Don't go to the grocery store hungry, or you will likely come home with sugary things you wouldn't normally buy.

Be mindful when you eat and enjoy every bite.

Peptides That Improve Metabolism and Decrease Sugar Cravings

IGF-1/CJC1295 and Ipamorelin

Remember when you were a kid and could eat everything in sight and not gain a pound? That's because we have high levels of growth hormone as kids. The workhorse for growth hormone is IGF-1, and this is a peptide that can help diminish sugar cravings. IGF-1 receptors are 600 times more prevalent than insulin receptors in the body and are your number one fat-burning hormone that stabilizes blood sugar spikes and drops. No more sugar cravings.

CJC 1295 is a peptide we use in conjunction with IGF-1 so that your pituitary makes more growth hormone so that your body feels more satiated when eating and energized. This peptide also helps you increase muscle mass.

Ipamorelin helps balance out both growth hormone pathways in your pituitary gland. Its main function is to allow your body to express life-giving hormones by inhibiting somatostatin. Ipamorelin tames ghrelin (the hormone that triggers food cravings), and it increases the effectiveness of the growth hormone spike by seven times when used with CJC 1295.

Energy Multiplier

Some of the herbs that can be used in conjunction with peptides are berberine, gymnema, and banaba. Each of these ingredients supports greater blood sugar stabilization for optimizing energy levels. Energy

Multiplier is a complete formula that will give your body the raw materials to support your blood sugar stability. You can find it at thesmartmedicine.com.

Chapter Five
Movement

Your Miracle Cure

Mindset Number Five
Moving your body daily is a gift that appreciates the more you use it.

Pop Quiz time: What therapy gives you a reduced risk of cardiovascular disease, cancer, and metabolic disease? This treatment provides mental and physical agility, stronger bones and muscles, and overall happiness.

You get improved functional mobility, higher self-esteem, better energy, great sleep, and less stress, depression, and anxiety.

Is this therapy for you? Any guesses as to what it is?

While there's no "magic bullet" for wellness, if we could bottle up all the benefits of exercise into a pill, we would! (Although Peptides like MOTS-c and 5 amino 1-MQ do come close.)

I had my own transformation at a very young age, thanks to the magic of exercise. When I was ten years old, I was overweight for my height. I loathed running (even though I had been playing sports since I was five) and became so out of shape that I felt nauseous during timed miles in gym class.

Even though my parents got me involved in a wide variety of activities (dance, soccer, floor hockey, tennis, rollerblading, riding bikes, etc.), I ate terribly and watched a lot of TV during my downtime.

My diet consisted of PB&J sandwiches made on Wonder bread with a side of Capri Sun. McDonald's was my go-to dinner, and my favorite foods all had some form of cheese: cheeseburgers, fried cheese sticks, stuffed cheesy potato skins, and sausage, egg, and cheese biscuits. I was a poster child for what not to eat.

One day, I had one of my first major mindset resets that changed my life forever. I had just come home from another travel soccer game, not having been played by the coaches because I couldn't keep up with the other girls, and I felt defeated. My dad had a heart-to-heart with me, sharing how he had gotten out of shape on the school wrestling team after having Mono for a month, so he took up running to get back into shape.

Something inside of me shifted during that conversation from self-pity to anger, and I said to myself, "Enough is enough!" I turned to my dad at ten years old and said, "Will you buy me a treadmill?" Remember, I HATED running!! My dad, in good faith, believed in me, took me to Dick's Sporting Goods, and bought me that treadmill.

I started out only being able to huff and puff through five minutes at moderate speed, but I didn't give up. The fire had ignited in my spirit, and I wanted to prove to everyone, including myself, that I could lose weight and keep up with my soccer teammates.

Fast forward, and after cutting out junk foods, eating my Mom's home-cooked meals, and working my way up to hour-long runs on the treadmill without stopping, I lost 25 lbs. I'll never forget how that felt.

I had a new lease on life. I felt more confident. I could fit into clothes that were meant to be my size, and I loved back-to-school shopping. When I was still overweight, I dreaded the dressing room and everything not fitting me, having to buy the largest size available for petite girls.

My new confidence carried over into every area of my life. After discovering I loved to sing at my local church, I decided to try out for "Annie" at a community theatre and booked the lead role at age 13. I kept booking community theatre roles while simultaneously playing sports in high school, staying incredibly active. I made the JV soccer team and ran varsity cross-country, lettered my freshmen year, was the third or fourth top runner on the team, and supported our team to the regional championship.

I truly thought, only so many years prior, that I would never get the chance to proudly wear a Mayfield Wildcat Letter Jacket around my high school because I wasn't "athletic enough".

Whenever your mind tells you you can't do something, it doesn't mean you can't. It just means at that moment you are believing a lie. Looking back, the moments in my life where I went from "I can't" to "I can" was all it took to shift my energy and get me to take action. I truly believe that resetting our mindset can have such a profound effect on how we approach anything in our lives. Thanks to my shift with exercise, I have continued to reap so many rewards for the past 23 years.

How is it that exercise is so powerful, it can transform your life? We're excited to share the answer, but first, some important statistics on how exercise is gravely underutilized as a habit.

With 70% to 80% of adults considered to be inactive and increasing rates of obesity, we actually might start seeing life expectancy decrease for the first time in generations.

The World Health Organization has listed physical inactivity as the fourth leading risk factor for early death.

According to the CDC, only 22% of Americans get enough exercise every day.

As published in the *Journal of Cardiovascular Research*: **Only 12% of Americans over the age of 20 are metabolically healthy.**

This generally means they have ideal levels of blood sugar, blood pressure, and cholesterol and do not take medications for these risk factors.

New research and decades of existing evidence suggest working out helps keep these factors in check. Researchers reveal that exercise sets off a cascade of metabolic changes and reprograms the way our bodies burn fuel.

Do these stats and studies surprise you? If everyone knew what a phenomenal treatment exercise could be, one could assume these numbers wouldn't be so low for exercise!

On a side note, did you know that the Wim Hoff breathing you learned will make it easier for you to exercise? Cutting out sugar will also tremendously reduce inflammation, giving you more energy for workouts, helping reduce aches and pains, and increasing how fast you recover. (We put these in order for a reason!)

Here's another very interesting study. A researcher named O'Sullivan and his team recruited 52 healthy soldiers newly enlisted to the Australian army. All the soldiers were around 26 years old with a healthy body mass index or healthy weight relative to height.

With this unique cohort, researchers got the chance to control potential confounding factors, elements that might sway the results like diet, stress levels, and work environment. All the soldiers ate the same food, kept the same sleep patterns, lived together, and performed the same daily activities.

The soldiers each completed the same mixed aerobic and strength exercise program for 80 days. They also completed strength and endurance workouts as well as traditional occupational activities related to the military, like marching. The researchers took blood samples before and after the participants completed the exercise program. Sixty-eight percent of the activity was moderate intensity, while 32% was high intensity.

After completing the exercise regimen, participants showed changes to numerous metabolites thought to positively influence immune function, increase blood flow, and fight inflammation, including the metabolites ARG, ORN, and I3P, which are all pro-inflammatory.

Participants experienced positive changes in other metabolites involved in blood clotting, the opening of blood vessels, the breakdown of protein, and stress reduction. The group showed "highly significant" changes across other metabolic compounds like lipids, ketone bodies, endocannabinoids, and nucleotides.

Participants' trained, energy-efficient muscles also shifted. Post-exercise, participants used far more fuel like fat and ketone bodies, as shown by a reduction of plasma, fatty acid, and ketone body intermediates in the blood.

For the first time, the true magnitude and extent of metabolic adaptation to chronic exercise training are revealed in this carefully designed study, which can be leveraged for novel therapeutic strategies in cardiometabolic disease.

Do you have physical barriers to exercise? We understand and love to help our patients get back to doing what they love, pain-free! We provide physical therapy, chiropractic work, acupuncture, and the best functional medicine treatments available to reduce pain and increase mobility.

While many of these habits aren't high impact, if you are hurting and itching to get back to doing physical activities, please contact us. If you aren't close enough to come to one of our clinics, we do offer remote support, or we can point you in the right direction.

The great news is all of these habits you are learning can positively impact your ability to exercise, and your ability to exercise positively impacts these habits as well!

The Difference Exercise Makes

Are you leading a sedentary lifestyle?

Let's take a side-by-side look at what a difference it makes when an individual exercises vs. when they are sedentary. (This is based on averages from a 40-year old exerciser vs. someone who does little to no physical activity. Sources include CDC, WebMD, *Men's Journal*, Harris Training Systems, and ABC News.)

THE DIFFERENCE EXERCISE MAKES

SEDENTARY		REGULAR EXERCISE
56% Sleep Well	**Sleep Quality**	83% Sleep Well
60-80 Beats Per Minute	**Ave. HR**	40-60 Beats Per Minute
Women <25 Men <30	**Max O2 Uptake**	Women 46-50 Men 48-53
Women 1600-2000/Day Men 2000-2600/Day	**Ave. Calories**	Women 2000-2400/Day Men 2000-2600/Day
Ave. American Lifespan 78.7 years	**Life Expectancy**	About 4 Years Longer
Sweat Less Efficiently	**Sweat**	Start Sweating Sooner

- Better Sleep? Check
- Better cardiovascular health? Check
- Live longer AND get to eat more calories? Sign me up!
- These are more of the many benefits of exercise!
- Lowered risk of early death by 40%!
- Prevention of weight gain
- Lowered risk of Colon Cancer by 60%!
- Lowered risk of Breast Cancer by 50%!
- Lowered risk of High Blood Pressure by about 40%
- Improved cardiorespiratory and muscular fitness
- Reduced Depression risk
- Lower Type II Diabetes risk by about 58%

You only need 150 to 200 minutes per week to get these benefits. That's just 20 to 30 minutes a day!

Exercise and the Immune System

Exercise supports the immune system in beautiful ways, and we need that system to support us now more than ever.

Regular moderate exercise decreases the inflammatory response and increases immune regulation. Exercise helps move and flush pathogens out of your airways and causes antibodies and white blood cells to circulate more rapidly and to the farthest reaches of your vascular system.

It also reduces the release of the stress hormone cortisol. Elevated cortisol inhibits your immune system. As mentioned in the Stress chapter, cortisol is meant to be higher in the morning, but there's a healthy range. We test this for our patients, so they know the best time of day for their body to exercise!

You don't want cortisol too high or too low. When cortisol is too high, growth hormone drops, and you don't get as much benefit from exercise. When it's too low in the morning upon waking, you may feel exhausted and have trouble getting out of bed. Cortisol isn't something to be eradicated but rather in alignment with circadian rhythms, which you'll learn about in the next chapter.

The temporary increase of body temperature with exercise may also weaken or kill certain bacteria or viruses (similar to your body's fever response).

Here are some examples of great exercise/movement routines to try.

Tabata

Tabata is twenty seconds of high-intensity movement followed by 10 seconds of rest, for even just eight rounds, four minutes total. Start slow and work your way up to longer Tabata workouts for 20 minutes, and you'll feel it.

This was created by Japanese scientist Dr. Izumi Tabata from research he conducted with his team from the National Institute of Fitness and Sports at Kagoshima Prefecture, Japan. Dr. Tabata found that it yields the most benefits in the shortest amount of time. It's a type of HIIT workout or High-Intensity Interval Training.

Hop on a fitness app or go to YouTube, search "Tabata workouts", and give it a try! You can also find bodyweight Tabata workout routines with a quick Google search.

Here's a sample:

Tabata Training: High Intensity all-out 20 seconds, then rest 10 seconds. Complete all four moves 20 seconds on, 10 seconds off, in a row. Go back to the beginning and repeat once for a four-minute workout, repeat four times for an eight-minute workout. Ten times through is 20 minutes, and so on!

- Squat Jumps
- Push-ups
- Burpees
- Sit-ups

Super-Slow Strength Training

This is a strength training technique in which you lift and lower a weight more slowly than usual. For example, you may take about 10 seconds to lift the weight and another 10 seconds to lower the weight. The goal of super-slow strength training is to limit momentum.

Sprints!

This is one of the best ways to boost brain-derived nootropic factors. Try a routine where you make a 30-

second sprint followed by a functional movement routine like burpees, dumbbell presses, alternating lunges, jumping rope, or jumping jacks. Do 30-second sprints in between each exercise you choose to do, and you'll be amazed at your results!

Doing slower movements in between sprints while still moving your body is a way of doing "active recovery", so you aren't going from sprints to stationary.

I (Anne) have experienced the benefit of sprints. Not only did I have to perform sprint drills for soccer and track growing up, but in college, I kept up with running, doing treadmill workouts in the gym. I found that I could do just a 20- to 30-minute routine on the treadmill where I'd do sprints for a short period of time, then moderate jog or run, and kept alternating. This made the workout go by much faster, and I got WAY more benefit for fat burning and stoking my metabolism than I would get just running or jogging at the same pace for the same duration of time, no intervals.

Additional great forms of exercise include:

- Bodyweight workouts (There are apps, online videos, and classes where you just use gravity and functional movements, no equipment necessary.)
- Strength/weight training (Start with a trainer/class instructor to prevent injury from improper form.)
- Running (Stretching is important! If you need to do movements that are not high impact, try an elliptical machine, biking, or swimming!)
- Peloton/Spin classes or outdoor biking

- Hiking, kayaking, and other outdoor sports
- Workout from home with your favorite YouTube video
- Dancing
- Get a Personal Trainer (This is fantastic for when you are brand new and definitely helps teach proper form and accountability.)
- Try Boxing
- Yoga
- High-Intensity Interval Training classes. Our team has classes we provide live and over video replay! No equipment necessary. We teach patients how to use props from home-like chairs and soup cans.
- Other classes (There are so many different styles and group fitness cultures. Do a Google search in your local area, and you'll be surprised what you find! ClassPass offers a way to find a wide variety of classes and try them out before buying full packages/membership. It's also great if you love constant variety.)
- Join a sports league like basketball, soccer, pickleball, tennis, etc.
- Pilates

Things to Keep in Mind

Walking and stretching are also really important. If you can't do any of the above routines due to illness or injury, do your best to walk and move every day as much as you can. Don't sit for long periods of time as you'll create tension, tightness, muscle atrophy, weakness, etc.

If you feel completely burnt out/have no energy, that may be a sign your adrenals are shot.

Remember the Stress chapter? This is when doing gentle recovery like yoga, walking, biking, etc., can be very supportive while you build yourself back up. Also, make sure to schedule your workout during a time of day that works in conjunction with your cortisol levels, which can be measured.

If you think you have little energy, but you notice lacing up your shoes and committing to your routine gives you energy once you're in action, then you are most likely not burnt out!

Sometimes mental fatigue makes us believe we don't have energy when that's the time we need to get moving! I once got home after a long day of work and thought I was tired, but my roommates put music on, started dancing in the living room, and suddenly, I had mountains of energy to spare!

Working out shouldn't feel like a chore! Find the routine that brings you the most joy, feels good in your body, challenges you in healthy ways, and is a sustainable habit.

If this feels intimidating at all, start low and slow. Even if it's just, "I will do crunches and pushups for five minutes each day," don't go from zero to 60 too fast.

It's also really important to get guidance in the beginning when you are brand-new to a workout routine that requires some form and technique. Speak to a trainer, or contact us. We have physical therapists and chiropractors who are obsessed with functional movement and want to help.

This is also the perfect time to put Habit Building 101 into place. Make sure, when starting your daily workout routine, you have the following. (Trust us, this works.)

- Have it written in your calendar and choose a specific time, whether it's a class or time you need to set aside for yourself to do an at-home routine. If you just say, "I'll work out," it's far less likely to happen. Book it.
- Have an accountability partner. This really helps you show up for yourself and is a lot more fun.
- Community. If you are someone who thrives on workouts in a group setting, there are great ways to create a sense of community and camaraderie with your exercise routine. You can find clubs that go on group hikes, join a sports league, find a gym that offers group social outings as a part of their culture, like circuit training gyms or Crossfit. There are even gyms and classes that blast great music and have fun lights while you work out, so you feel like you're at a party!

Challenge for the Week

We're going to do this in tiers.

For beginners, your goal is to exercise a bare minimum of eight minutes per day. Remember the "Make it easy" part of habit building? This is it. If you aren't ready for 30, start here and work your way up. If your brain is still resisting eight minutes, say to yourself, "I'll do two minutes," and once you get going, the hardest part is over!

The next level is 22 minutes. Just 22 minutes, including warmup and cooldown, leaves about 16 minutes of moderate work. Your favorite television shows are about that long, not including commercials. Do your workout during your show and see how time flies!

Ideal Goal: Do 30 minutes of moderate exercise every single day. Try some of the sample workouts we've recommended!

***Bonus Points:**

Exercise outdoors and get fresh air and sunshine!

Give yourself a personal challenge! For example, find a half-marathon or 5k and give yourself a training schedule with a deadline. If you are already light years ahead of us with this challenge, we commend you. Give yourself a new challenge that pushes you in ways that excite you.

Signing up for a competition or race of some kind where you are competing against yourself and giving yourself healthy goals is a terrific way to establish new motivation and get something on the calendar.

Don't forget to give yourself recovery time. We don't want you working out at your max intensity every single day. Even Olympic athletes need proper recovery. Choose a couple of days a week when you'll work out more intensely, two or three days for a moderate workout, and a couple of low-impact stretching and recovery days with activities like yoga and walking, hiking, taking a bike ride, etc. Your body benefits greatly from variety, and you'll never be bored!

Bonus Resources

Here are some books Regan loves!

Younger Next Year by Chris Crowley

Research has shown that, as we age, we need greater exercise. They recommend 60 to 90 minutes every day. Now, that's a great goal to work up to once you nail your Challenge!

Body by Science by Dr. Doug McGuff

This is a great book if you are looking to learn strength training through super slow movements (as mentioned above) without putting extra pressure on your joints and preventing injury. Look up his videos as well!

Are you pumped to go work out? Put this book down, head out the door, and get moving!

Peptides for Workout Recovery, Stem Cell Health, and Muscle Building

Have you ever been really sore after a workout? Maybe it's two or three days after you really pushed yourself, but the leg tightness and muscle aches are hard to forget.

Thymosin Beta 4 is my go-to recovery peptide post-workout. It turns out it improves stem cell health in joints, removes metabolic waste from muscles, and supports connective tissue, skin, and helps improve immunity. You can get a fragment of this made by my friend and colleague Kent Holtorf, MD, called TB4 FRAG, and see if it doesn't help.

Optimal Movement

While exercise can break down muscles and supportive structures, collagen is the nutrient that rebuilds your stronger skeletal system. The Optimal Movement formula is a great way to get the right kind of collagen support that your body can easily digest, but it also helps tame the inflammation from your workout. Try it for yourself at thesmartmedicine.com

Chapter Six
Sleep

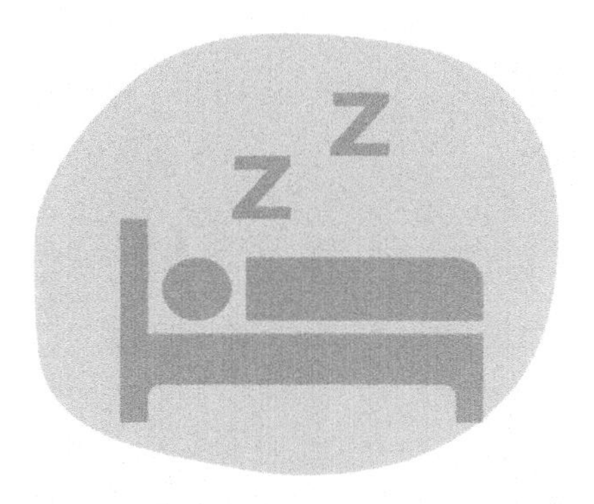

The Passive HAC to Feel Amazing

Mindset Number Six
You set high sleep standards so you can enjoy consistent energy levels.

> *"Lack of sleep induces critical changes within the brain, altering behavior and emotions, while also disturbing essential metabolic processes and influencing the expression of immune-related genes. The end result is that people who are sleep-deprived avoid social interaction."* ~Dr. Matthew Walker, author of *Why We Sleep*

I learned this valuable lesson the hard way after years of depriving myself of the joy and many benefits of sleep.

When I was in high school, I didn't understand the importance of sleep, and man, I wish that I had! My test scores may have been quite different for my SATs and ACTs. I did well enough but had no idea how much sleep affects brainpower.

I was so exhausted from school, then after-school sports and rehearsals, then doing homework late into the night that I'd have to leave school early some days to take a nap before heading right back to rehearsals for a show. I was always trying to "catch up", not knowing that you can't catch up from a poor sleep routine. And those three-hour "cat naps" left me in a dazed and confused state until the performance adrenaline kicked in.

My sleep habits even led me to stay up until 3 am and sleep in until noon on weekends, wasting half the day away with my room darkening curtains pulled down tight. Even as I type this, I'm amazed at how awful my sleep routine was and how I let it get so bad.

I carried this poor habit with me to college, where I would stay up until 1 am working on class assignments, get up at

7 am for early morning ballet class, and then went non-stop all day.

College was where I discovered the joys of caffeine that allowed me to quiet my body's ability to tell me I'm tired and made me feel superhuman all day long. I'd crash in the afternoons and crave sugar, so I'd grab a pick-me-up and keep ongoing.

During exam weeks, I was stressed to the max, trying to keep up with academics and my freshman year Musical Theatre major. Though I told myself I'd never do this, I pulled an all-nighter to write a 12-page paper. I'm so grateful I didn't succumb to things like Adderall and become addicted.

Eventually, I did gain the dreaded "Freshman 15" and thought it was strictly my diet and exercise that were to blame. I also caught every cold and flu on campus that would wipe me out for several days, where I'd finally allow myself the joy of sleep to recover. It was only when I was sick that I thought I had "earned the right to rest."

Come senior year of college, I had another "enough is enough" moment. I had become very interested in health and was reading every article I could find on food and fitness when I learned the importance of getting seven to eight hours of quality sleep per night. It finally hit me that all those years of pushing through exhaustion in high school and college had led me to deplete my body of an essential habit. All that I needed to change was to "permit" myself to sleep!

I was in control of my schedule, so why wasn't I letting myself go to bed earlier? My perfectionist-overachieverproductivity-obsessed side wouldn't allow it. I was always feeling overwhelmed with the amount I wanted to get done, and I felt a jolt of creative energy hit me around 11:30 pm every night and would strike while the iron was hot.

When I started giving myself a set bedtime of midnight and wake time of 8 am, it was a game-changer. I credit sleep coupled with dietary changes for also boosting my immune system immensely. I was no longer catching every bug that went around, and I felt so much better from adequate recovery.

I tell you this story so that, if you are like I was in college, you will stop and start to question what "reasoning" you may be giving yourself for why you are depriving yourself of sleep. That is, of course, unless you are a parent, in which case I salute you and completely understand the struggle is so real.

Did you know that we can go longer without food than we can without sleep? Deficient sleep not only increases the chances of you getting sick it also prolongs your recovery.

In some instances, lack of sleep can literally lead to death. Take this story, for example. This 26-year-old stayed up for 11 days bingeing televised soccer games and very sadly, ended up dead from exhaustion: www.huffpost.com/entry/man-dies-11-days-no-sleep-deprivation

Sleeping less than five hours per night doubles the risk of death from cardiovascular disease. That's the number one killer in America, currently.

While some have proven that they can stay awake 11 days straight and not lose their lives, they are doing a lot of damage in the process.

Examples of the damage include:

- Blood sugar irregularities
- Sugar cravings
- Moodiness
- Ghrelin (your hunger hormone causing you to overeat)
- Low performance
- Brain fog
- Anger/hostility
- Confusion
- Likelihood of getting sick
- Likelihood of potential disease onset
- Likelihood of making mistakes or getting into accidents (fatal car accidents increase by 6% on average each year during Daylight Savings Time: www.healthline.com/health-news/daylight-saving-can-make-driving-less-safe#Fatal-car-accidents-spike-when-we-spring)

Sleep has proven to improve and sustain a vast array of functions, including cellular immunity, reproduction, cognition, cardiovascular, and other health functions. Your body also produces and releases cytokines when you sleep. Cytokines are proteins that target inflammation.

The point is that ***quality sleep matters***.

What does quality sleep look like?

Science says seven to eight hours of sleep per night is needed for optimal health, but this can vary from person to person. If you are waking up feeling well-rested, that is a good marker.

Think of a time in your life when you slept best. What were you doing to help you wake up feeling refreshed?

We'll be teaching you "Sleep Hygiene" techniques that can help you have your best night's sleep. There are many available now to help you biohack your way to the best rest possible.

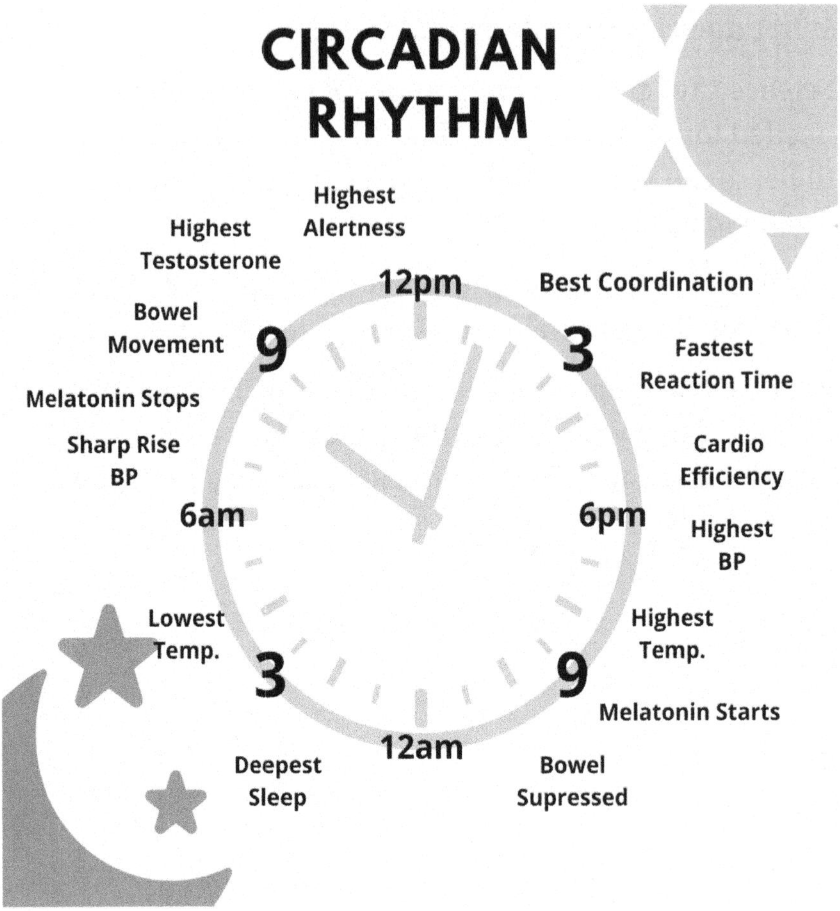

CIRCADIAN RHYTHM

Highest Alertness

Highest Testosterone

12pm

Best Coordination

Bowel Movement

9

3

Fastest Reaction Time

Melatonin Stops

Sharp Rise BP

Cardio Efficiency

6am

6pm

Highest BP

Lowest Temp.

Highest Temp.

3

9

Melatonin Starts

12am

Deepest Sleep

Bowel Supressed

Above is an infographic on the different phases of the day and what your body is naturally going through. Along with the above graph, we encourage you to look at the "Horary" time clock, which shows, in Traditional Chinese Medicine, the specific times of day that are aligned with certain organs in the body.

Working in conjunction with this natural rhythm and doing activities in alignment with it helps you stay in the flow with nature and ultimately makes life easier by living as nature intended.

For example, in seeing that the graph shows melatonin starting to kick in around 9 pm, that's not the time to be doing stimulatory activities and confusing your body, nor pushing through and staying up late to watch your favorite show. We ideally should be going to bed between nine and 10 pm at the latest to follow what the body is doing: getting us ready for sleep!

Putting priority tasks earlier in the day when we are most alert, mid-morning, can help us feel much more productive. For some, exercising first thing in the morning as cortisol raises you up is also helpful to start the day feeling calm rather than diving right into work or drinking coffee, feeling high-strung.

This is also why, as you'll learn in the Timed Eating chapter, it's so important not to disrupt the processes that need to take place as you are sleeping. For example, eating too close to bedtime forces your body to focus on digesting the food as you lie down rather than the process of repair.

First thing in the morning, as you wake up, let your body breathe. That being said, don't keep hitting snooze. Just let your body come out of the restful state. Allow dreams to come to your consciousness if they do. Dreams may give you some guidance.

In mid-afternoon, you have your greatest coordination and fastest reaction time if you are able to do a physical activity.

This also shows you why NOT to test your blood pressure, if you need to monitor it, later in the evening around 6 pm as that's the time of day your body's blood pressure is naturally higher.

Social media scrolling (dopamine hit) or passively watching TV shows or movies that make your heart race and perk up your brain are not ideal activities in the evening. Be conscious of your media consumption, especially as you wind down to sleep.

We've provided a step-by-step plan for how to utilize Sleep Hygiene and get the best night's sleep of your life every night!

Sleep Hygiene 101:

1. In the morning, give yourself some time in the sun without sunglasses on.
2. Stop caffeine by 9 am and decaf teas or coffee by 12 pm. Caffeine can take 12 hours to metabolize, and decaf still has some leftovers as the caffeine has to be processed out.

3. Follow the Circadian Rhythm chart above and seek to do activities in conjunction with nature and the time of day that is best. For example, 10 am to 2 pm is your most productive time of day for getting priorities taken care of.
4. If you feel wired at night and tired in the morning when cortisol should be helping you rise, get a salivary cortisol test to see if your levels are off.
5. Discover your ideal time to work out in alignment with the clock and your cortisol levels.
6. Stop eating at least three hours before your bedtime. This allows time to fully digest your food. Otherwise, it can severely throw off your body's ability to optimally sleep and detox at night. You shouldn't go to bed feeling shaky or starving, so find the window that is best for you.
7. Don't do an intense workout before bed. That can throw your natural circadian rhythms off.
8. No screen time at least one, preferably two hours before bed. This includes blue light-producing screens like TVs, phones, smart tablets, etc. If you have to utilize any of those devices close to bedtime, wear blue-light-blocking glasses. You can snag a pair online at Amazon.
9. Instead of screen time, which not only disrupts you from the blue light but also can excite the nervous system like checking e-mail or watching a horror film, choose a relaxing activity or one that positively gives your brain something to do. Don't stress over a to-do list or ask your brain to process

complex information. Instead, try a light card game, a crossword puzzle, reading a book, etc. This is the ideal time to give your brain something to do.

10. Reddish hues are more calming in the evening, blocking the blue light.

11. If you are having anxious, racing thoughts, try a calming, deeply relaxing activity like an epsom salt bath, soothing binaural beats for sleep, herbal teas like chamomile, taking some magnesium, meditation, etc.

12. Set your room up for success. Try your best to keep the TV out of the bedroom to feel less tempted. Regan has said, "The bedroom is for sleep and sex." You can get high-quality pillows (keep them clean of bacteria and mold) and look into investing in a better quality mattress (there are many out there made from non-gas-producing materials that don't heat you up and are organic).

13. Keep your room between 65 and 70 degrees. You want your bedroom cool. You can buy what Regan uses to keep himself very cool and doesn't disrupt his partner, which is a "Chili Pad". If your body is too hot at night, that can disrupt your sleep.

14. It's ideal to go to bed between nine and 10 pm at the latest, as your body doesn't hit deeper REM sleep (Rapid Eye Movement) until further into your sleep cycle. You don't want to disrupt that with the sunrise.

The Mindset Morning

This is something Regan does every day and recommends to each of his patients to start their day on the best note possible:

- Meditate and/or pray for five minutes, whatever practice gets you in touch with your deeper calm.
- Write down and reflect on your goals for five minutes.
- Write down anyone you would like to reach out to.
- Visualize all of the above goals actualized for five minutes.
- Brush your teeth, wash your face, and make your bed every single day.
- Exercise.

Challenge Time: Track Your Sleep!

You can download free apps or just track your sleep on a sheet of paper each night. You can also buy devices now that will track your sleep in greater detail if that interests you, but it's not a requirement. Plan on doing your mindset morning above, and based on your current routine, tweak at least one of your sleep hygiene tools above that could make for the best quality sleep possible. After these 100 days, you'll be amazed how much your entire sleep routine has changed for the better!

Peptides that Are "Deep Sleep Inducing"

DSIP (Deep Sleep Inducing Peptides) can retrain your pineal gland to express the right amount of melatonin at the right time. Sometimes, we DO need some help getting to and staying asleep. This is a sleep-inducing peptide that induces delta brain waves. It works on the pineal gland to stabilize melatonin, serotonin, and oxytocin levels.

Chapter Seven
Water

Are You Hydrated?

Mindset Number Seven
You first take care of hydration with proper electrolytes and quantities of pure water to nourish your cells.

"Water is the softest thing, yet it can penetrate mountains and earth. This shows clearly the principle of softness overcoming hardness."
~Laozi

Water is yet another undervalued, underutilized resource to your best health.

Whether you are someone who doesn't drink enough water, believe you drink enough yet still aren't "hydrating" your body, or possibly even someone who drinks too much water, this information will finally give you all the guidance you need on optimal hydration!

Why is water so important? What does it actually do for us?

Water Has Seven Key Functions in the Body:

- Transports all of the hormones, peptides, nutrients, waste products, and genetic functions.
- Dissolves and breaks down solids, including things like kidney stones.
- Cleans your kidneys as well as your liver as a filtration system. Your ability to detox depends on water.
- Helps get hormones and neurotransmitters where they need to go and supports conductivity.
- Pads joints. Did you know we are shorter by the end of the day?? Think of the discs in your spine like water-filled jelly donuts. If you don't have

enough water to pad those discs, they compress, and you, quite literally, shrink.

- Regulates body temperature.

What happens when we're dehydrated?

For one, your chance of becoming obese is one and a half times greater if you are chronically dehydrated!

Water makes up 60% of your body. Just 2% loss of water causes physical performance and mental cognition to decrease by 20 to 40% depending on the temperature!

Your brain is 75% water, blood is 92% water, muscles are 75% water, and bones are 22% water. The percentage of water on the planet is about the same as the amount of water in our bodies! Personally, I don't think that's a coincidence. Our bodies are the microcosm of the macrocosm.

Dehydration can lead to less motor function and short-term memory loss. It even impacts your mood and can create exhaustion, anxiety, and greater negative thinking if you are depleted.

It even affects your skin, leading to preventable wrinkles and dryness.

Water has all of these benefits, yet three out of four Americans are dehydrated.

While thirst would seemingly be a good indicator for whether or not you have had enough water, that actually means you may already be dehydrated. It's ideal to drink throughout the day, consistently, *before* you become thirsty.

While the general consensus is that we need an average of 10 glasses a day, needs vary person to person depending on activity level, how much you sweat, climate, etc.

Do You Know How Dehydrated You Are in the Morning?

You are eight to 12 ounces dehydrated by the time you wake up. Check out your urine. If it's dark, you are dehydrated. If you aren't peeing at all, you are *really* dehydrated.

First thing in the morning, you need one or two glasses of clean filtered water with minerals to replenish.

Soda, coffee, sports drinks, and alcohol can lead to further dehydration. I'm sorry to disappoint you, and I'm sure you can find on Google where you're told the opposite, but coffee and caffeinated beverages do not "count" in your daily water intake.

They are diuretics, meaning they make you urinate more frequently and can deplete and diminish nutrient levels. For every one cup or eight ounces of coffee or caffeine, drink that same amount of pure water on top of your daily intake. Alcohol requires two glasses of water for every one alcoholic drink you have.

The types of sodium and potassium in things like Gatorade can actually further dehydrate rather than support you! That type of potassium causes your body to want more, so your body starts sloughing off chloride.

That was wild for me to learn from Regan, as I had grown up being told to "drink a Gatorade" if I needed to replenish electrolytes from exercise or even when sick. Gatorade is chock full of sugar, dyes, and other fake sweeteners. It's really not a supportive health drink at all.

Having 4700 mg of potassium daily is not only important for hydration and eliminating excess water weight, but you'll also learn in chapter 12 how it affects blood sugar transport into your cells!

Water and Fat Burning

Simply being hydrated can activate your body's ability to burn fat like a well-watered machine.

Water activates the transportation of these Six Fat Burning Hormones:

1. Thyroid Hormones (T3 and T4)
2. Growth Hormone (GH)
3. Insulin-Like Growth Factor (IGF-1)
4. Testosterone
5. Glucagon
6. Adrenaline

If you are dehydrated, your fat cells become greedy, hungry machines sending out inflammatory signals. The fat cells then don't allow water to get into the cells where it needs to go.

In this case, we need optimal minerals, not just water. Adequate levels of healthy, positively charged sodium can lead to optimal hydration as it helps shuttle water into the cell.

Optimal hydration of the cells allows Growth Hormone to come in and do its job. (On a side note, you can actually take peptides that stimulate growth hormone, which further helps water get into the cell, boosting hydration. That's provided at the end of this chapter.)

Getting water into the cell helps reduce bloat from water weight and retention.

Too much sugar circulating in the blood will also lend itself to weight gain. Being properly hydrated can fix this. Making sure you are properly hydrating before jumping on a blood sugar-regulating supplement regimen can be greatly beneficial.

You have 600 times more receptor cells for IGF-1 than you do for insulin. IGF-1 helps your body grow and repair, burns fat and helps you gain muscle. Optimal hydration allows this to be released from the liver.

A study was conducted to show the impact of water intake for men and women between the ages of 55 and 75 years old who were overweight or obese (BMI between 25 and 40 kg/m^2).

Researchers excluded recent yo-yo dieters. That meant the participants' weight had to be the same, within two kilograms (about five pounds) for the last year or longer. Before the study started, everyone had to come into the lab twice: once to eat as much food as they wanted, and once to drink 500 mL of water and *then* eat as much as they wanted.

Researchers wanted to see whether people would eat less if they drank water before a meal. Twelve weeks later, at the end of the study, the participants did the water-drinking test again.

Conclusion

Drinking water (500 mL or about 16 oz, which equates to two cups) *before* three meals a day while on a diet increases fat loss in overweight and obese individuals.

By drinking 500 mL of water, your body would use 24% more calories for 60 minutes after drinking water!

This is due to changes in osmolarity caused by drinking water and that your body has to expend energy to bring everything back in balance.

You'd be amazed how quickly you'll lose weight just from getting hydrated.

I realized this quickly in college when I'd eat a full dinner but still feel hungry afterward. It turns out, the signal for hunger can be confused with thirst. To test this, I drank two glasses of water after dinner, and voilà, I felt full. By increasing my water intake throughout the day to prevent dehydration later on, I was able to eat a normal size dinner and feel satiated.

Stress

If you are drinking enough water, with minerals, and still feeling puffy, stress could be the culprit! It can throw off your mineral levels despite your best efforts.

That's where working with a functional medicine provider comes in handy. They can help you decipher where the stressors may be coming from. These stressors represent the "4" in our "3-4-5 Method" of healing.

Just remember the acronym E.P.I.C which stands for Emotional, Physical, Immune, or Chemical. The providers can also check to see if your stress hormones are off, as well as many other markers of good health.

Organs and Systems Dependent on Water

Digestion

Since water stimulates movement, it makes sense that dehydration would cause constipation.

At the same time, too much water in the system actually puts a burden on the kidneys and flushes minerals out, causing you to become dehydrated, especially when the water you are drinking is "dead water" without minerals, like distilled water. Animals fed distilled mineral-free water will die after only two months.

You must replenish these minerals once water is filtered. This includes magnesium, potassium, sodium, etc. This can easily be done with a high-quality mineral supplement added back to your clean water like Trace Mineral brand, Redmond's Sea Salt, Quinton Essentials, etc.

Skin

Dehydrated skin lacks water, feels oily and dry at the same time, and is prone to breakouts. Do you want to up your skin regimen? Start by making sure you are hydrated internally before moving immediately to all the topical products available (so many of which have chemicals that are not ideal for skin absorption).

Joints

Your joints contain bursa sacs filled mostly with water. When you jump, punch, fall, or even move, these sacs prevent the ends of the two bones from smashing into one another.

Between the vertebrae of your spine, water makes up the filling of your vertebral discs that allow you to bend, twist and jump without agony. Just ask someone with degenerative back disease how important it is to have water in your discs.

Water can help with degenerative knees, discs, etc. If you don't have enough water, your cushioning from the bursa sacs can wear out, and you no longer have that support. There will be more pressure on your knees, back, shoulders, and more.

Muscles

Hydration can reduce lactic acid buildup and cramping! If you are super tight, it could be yet another sign you need better hydration.

Fluoride in Your Water

A study was done in Iran showing the effects of fluoride in regular drinking water on the thyroid gland. [*Scientific Reports*, 2018 (Feb 8)]

It was found that the elevated fluoride in water, when consumed, negatively impacted T3, T4, and TSH levels.

This problem remains unsolved, even with the addition of iodine in salt.

The application of standard household water purification (such as reverse osmosis, electrodialysis, activated carbon filter, and other adsorption/ion-exchange methods) is recommended for patients with hypothyroidism and those dealing with thyroid imbalances. The purification systems can help remove fluoride that interferes with thyroid functions.

Fluoride is also a stabilizer for drugs. Pharmaceutical companies were allowed to dump the waste product on land, which later ended up in conventional drinking water. This has impacted farming animals as well as people.

100,000,000 Cells Die Every Single Minute

If you are hydrated, the stem cells replacing those dead cells need hydration. Cells need the fluid to help nutrients populate the cell.

We replace our skin cells every 28 days, liver cells every 500 days, intestinal cells every three days, white blood cells every few hours, and red blood cells every 120 days.

This is why we read Hemoglobin A1C as a measure for blood sugar through the red blood cells since they last a little longer than three months!

CD34 cells are the most populous stem cells and are located in your small intestines. Hence, gut health is so important, as is removing inflammation in your small intestines.

Nutrients and oxygen, which are important for the cell to grow and repair itself, also depend on water.

Cell waste products, like carbon dioxide, need water to be eliminated from the system.

Water is an important molecule involved in most of the body's chemical reactions. In some cases, it has to be broken down or hydrolyzed during chemical reactions.

When sugar (sucrose) is digested into fructose and glucose, water is also a part of the reaction and is hydrolyzed.

How do you know you're dehydrated?

- Dehydration starts before you are even thirsty!
- Look at your urine, which should be light to clear. Take a look at the helpful infographic of colors below.
    - Don't worry. If it's neon yellow and you take B vitamins, that would be why.
- Spots on nails/cracks.
- Headaches.

- Muscle cramps.
- Red in urine or cloudiness could be indicative of kidney infection. Don't be dismissive! Get checked if you notice blood or cloudy urine right away.
- Strong smells. Did you know that if your pee smells like coffee, it's crappy coffee?! Buy it organic from a brand that also ensures there is no mold toxicity. Certain brands have high standards and test for mold.
- Get your labs done! Blood work can show your provider if you are truly hydrated or not.

URINE TEST

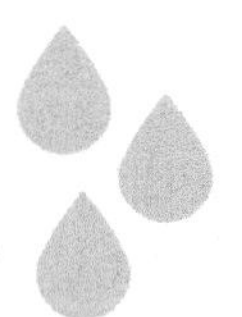

CHECK THE COLOR OF YOUR URINE BELOW TO SEE YOUR HYDRATION STATUS

TRANSPARENT

You may be drinking too much

PALE YELLOW

You're well hydrated!

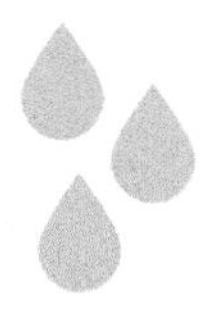

TRANSPARENT YELLOW

You're normal.

DARK YELLOW

You could use more water soon.

AMBER OR HONEY

You are dehydrated. Drink some water.

SYRUP OR BROWN ALE

You are severely dehydrated/may have liver issues. Consult a doctor.

LIGHT PINK OR RED

Did you eat beets, rhubard, or other red food? If not it could be blood or another issue. Consult a doctor.

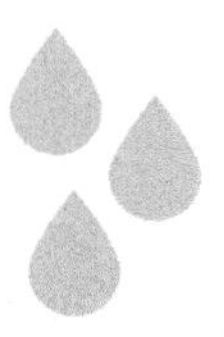

Three Steps to Proper Water Intake

Step 1: Remove Chemicals

There are way too many chemicals you'd never expect ending up in our groundwater: pesticides, medication byproducts, dry cleaning agents, and a lot more. Aquatru lists the 80+ chemicals removed by their reverse osmosis water filtration system alone.

Even before you increase your water intake, make sure your water is actually clean. While you may not be able to see a lot of the toxins in the water, go to www.ewg.org and look up the cleanliness of your local water. You might be surprised. Most tap water is not ideal for consumption in the U.S. You can also search for water filtration systems on the EWG.

AquaTru reverse osmosis is a great product you can look into as well. It pulls out chemicals, including glyphosate, which is a toxin found in RoundUp (a pesticide) used on the majority of non-organic crops and soils. This is so prevalent that even eating organic non-pesticide-ridden foods is not enough. We're all exposed to glyphosate.

Drinking water out of glass or stainless-steel water bottles is also preferred to plastics that can leach chemicals into the water you are drinking. Save your money and the planet, and buy reusable bottles and glasses from safe materials. Add in a water filtration system and calculate how much money you'll save by not buying water bottles daily/weekly!

Step 2: Add Electrolytes/Minerals

To accomplish this, you can add a pinch of Redmond's salt, Trace Minerals brand drops, or something like Quintessential brand for minerals. You'll feel the difference: less cramping, more energy, and you won't be peeing as much because the water is getting into the cells where it needs to be!

As mentioned, it's best to get your labs done and not just guess how much you need. It's not just about increasing, but it's important to have the right ratios of vitamins and minerals.

Don't add iodized table salt. In fact, throw that salt out and make sure you have a high-quality sea salt you are cooking with in general.

To make your water more interesting, add flavor naturally, and get additional benefits, you can try this detox drink below, or even add things to your water to infuse it like cucumber, mint, basil, strawberry, lemon, lime, and other fruits and herbs.

Ingredients:

8 oz spring water

2 oz unsweetened cranberry juice

1/3 fresh lemon juice or 1 tsp lemon powder. If you have a diagnosis of kidney stones, use the juice of a whole lemon or 3 tsp lemon powder.

½-1 tsp apple cider vinegar. Adjust to taste as this may be too strong for some people.

It is recommended that you mix the entire combination together in a container the night before and place it in the refrigerator or cooler.

Step 3: Track and Drink ~½ Your Body Weight in Ounces Per Day! (More if you sweat or are active a lot.)

Your Challenge:

- Buy a filter if you don't already have one. If you need to start with something simple like Britta, start there. No more tap water!
- Set a goal each day and see what feels best. Use your urine as an indicator. If you are noticing your urine is overly clear, you may be drinking too much, or you need more minerals.
- Start by drinking one or two glasses of water upon waking.
- Make sure to add minerals. Simply adding Redmond's salt is a good place to start.

- Notice the difference it's making! The more rewarding your habit, the more likely you are to stick with it consistently. Are you experiencing more energy? Glowing skin? Less brain fog? Take note!

Peptides for the Kidneys-ARA-290

Your kidneys are incredibly busy, and while ARA-290 has been shown to stabilize blood sugar Hemoglobin A1c levels, triglycerides, and cholesterol, it also works to promote erythropoietin, a hormone produced by the kidneys to create red blood cells.
pubmed.ncbi.nlm.nih.gov/25387363

I find that many patients who are chronically dehydrated also have anemic tendencies, kidney imbalances, and issues with cholesterol. ARA-290 is a lifesaver and if you happen to have any neuropathy in your feet or your hands. Studies show that this peptide helps heal the small nerve fibers that are damaged.

Chapter Eight
Cold

COLD

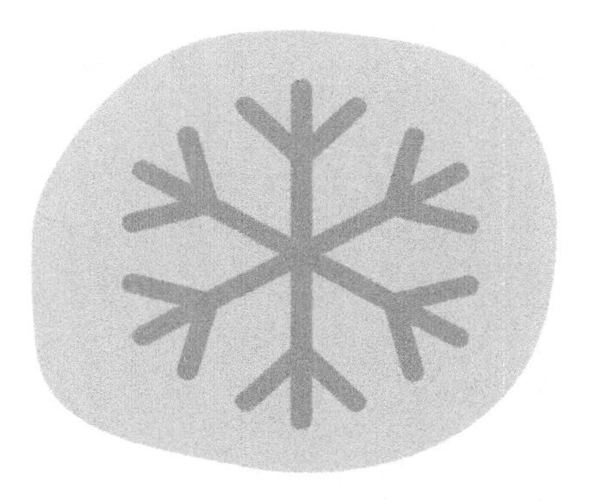

Freeze Your Troubles Away

Mindset Number Eight
Twenty seconds of cold for a leaner, more energized me? Sign me up! You are stronger than you give yourself credit for.

I can't believe we are halfway through!

Time for a check-in: How are you doing with these challenges? What are you noticing? What are your wins? Are you experiencing any resistance to change? Are there ways we can support these changes through your habit-building tools, mindset tools, and giving yourself some loving gratitude?

Write down what you have learned so far. Make sure to take time to celebrate yourself and how far you've come! Further challenges and difficulties are inevitable, but you are upleveling to be able to handle anything that comes your way. We celebrate you today and every day for your 1% gains.

Now, we've been building up week by week with foundations before we "plunge" into some biohacking techniques. (Pun intended.) This particular one is Regan's absolute favorite.

In 2020, on Regan's 42nd birthday, he decided to make an ice bath for himself to celebrate the beginning of his forty-second trip around the sun.

Lying in the ice and cold water wasn't easy, but after about three minutes, the endorphins kicked in, and he felt a deep sense of peace and relaxation that typically accompanies cold exposure.

He enjoyed the sensation so much that he decided to get into an ice bath every day until his next birthday, which he has since accomplished and surpassed. He enjoys it so much that on most summer days, he takes two baths!

The benefits of ice baths and cold exposure are enormous, but the biggest boost Regan gets out of it is mental clarity. It may sound crazy, but there are science-backed benefits to freezing your butt off.

Regan's co-host, partner, and brother, Cade, also enjoyed this process so much that he converted a meat freezer into an ice plunge! Cade will jump in his hot tub and back into his ice bath several times over to get all of the hormetic benefits of extreme temperature variations.

White Fat vs. Brown Fat

White fat is the type of fat you don't want. It increases TNF-α (tumor necrosis-alpha), inflammation, and insulin resistance. Too much white fat builds up in obese individuals. Its main role is to store fat and is more prevalent in the body than brown fat.

Brown fat, on the other hand, is the type of fat you *do* want. It breaks down blood glucose and fat molecules to create heat and helps maintain body temperature. It actively burns calories and energy.

With fat cells, the mitochondria in the center of the cell are "lazy". In order to get them metabolically functioning, we need to activate the mitochondria (the engines of your cells). When converted from white to brown adipose tissue, the fat cells become thermogenic. Cold therapy helps this thermogenic effect take place. The cold induces Brown Adipose Tissue activation and stimulates lipolysis, also known as fat burning.

When your brain is made aware and your body temperature comes down, you get an epinephrine and norepinephrine rush, then cortisol hits. This is your "stressed" state. Instead of waiting for sugar and protein to be released, cortisol tells fat cells to fuel and warm the body instead. This sympathetic nervous system response helps the liver and supports the conversion of T4 into T3 for the thyroid. The longer you do this, the quicker this process turns on.

A study looked at whether cold exposure could help the body use glucose in a more efficient fashion. Activating BAT (Brown Adipose Tissue) was shown to improve glucose homeostasis and increase energy expenditure. This is great news for diabetics! Pyruvate moves glucose into the cell, bypassing the need for insulin during cold exposure. Fatty acids get released into the bloodstream, shrinking your fat cells.
pubmed.ncbi.nlm.nih.gov/2667731

The best way to let it hit you is on the head and upper body, neck, and shoulder area during a cold shower. That's where most adults carry the most BAT!

While cold showers are perfect and free, you can also do what Cade Archibald has done and buy a meat freezer, creating your own cold tub without a large monetary investment. You can also dump ice into your bathtub and get the same effect.

Activating BAT and Thyroid Hormone

The BAT is mainly found in deposits located in the cervical-supraclavicular, perirenal/adrenal, and paravertebral regions. See the darker spots in the image below for reference.

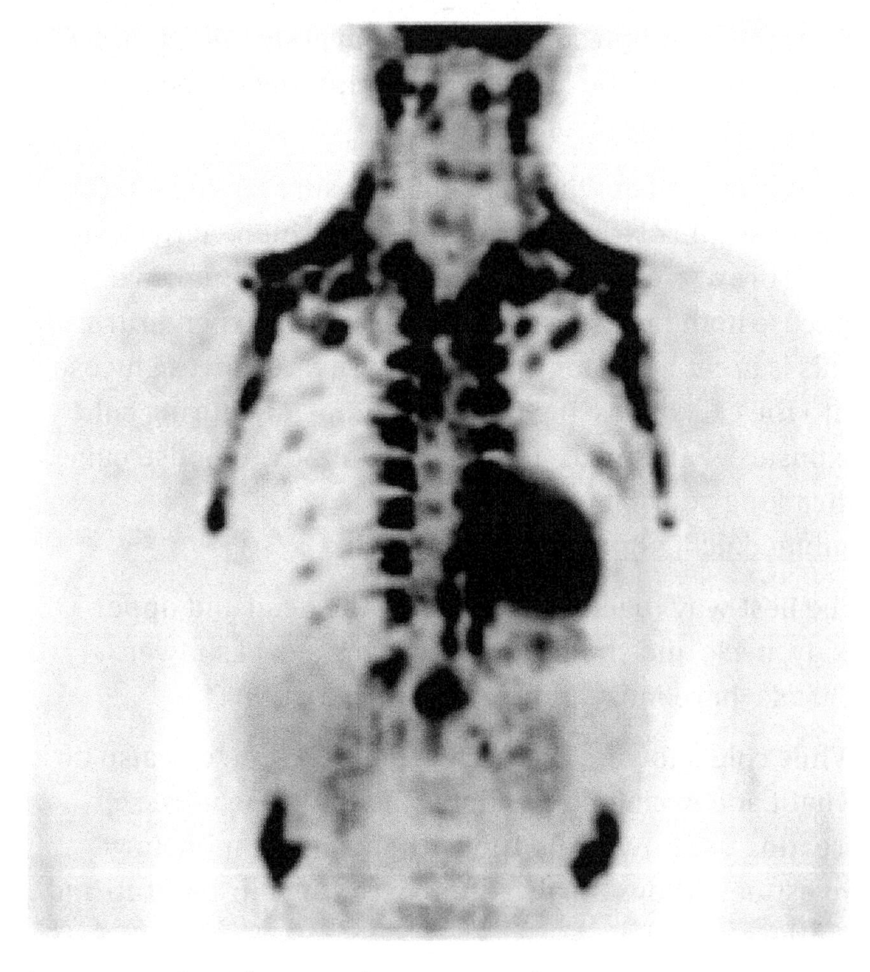

Image is taken from: pubs.rsna.org/

Cold exposure triggers a thermogenic program through the elevation of norepinephrine (secreted by neurons and alternatively activated macrophages) and thyroid hormone levels. Macrophages are cells involved in the detection and destruction of harmful organisms. This process also stimulates the immune system to become stronger.

BAT activation dissipates energy and activates heat. Your body is fighting to keep you warm. If you get exposed too long, you will go into hypothermia, which we do not want.

During cold exposure, your hands and feet are the first to feel very cold as the heat moves towards your internal organs. If you are doing an ice bath and want to last a little longer, you can stick your hands and feet outside the tub.

Cold and the Gut

Obesity is characterized by gut microbiota dysbiosis and reduced thermogenic activity of brown adipose tissue. A recent study reveals that gut microbiota hampers the emergence of thermogenic brown fat cells named beige cells within white fat deposits via a mechanism that involves the control of macrophages and eosinophil infiltration. The gut microbiota of obese individuals especially needs the support of cold exposure not only for insulin sensitivity but to counter this dampening effect of white fat conversion. (Nicholson J.K. "Host-gut microbiota metabolic interactions")

Thirty percent of the bacteria in your gut control your internal genetic "clock". Certain types of bacteria are more active at certain times of the day and are either storing or burning calories.

A study done by Claire Chevalier and colleagues from Geneva, Switzerland, published in *CELL*, not only shows that cold exposure (of mice) changes their gut microbes but also that, when transplanted into sterile mice, these "cold" microbes stimulate the formation of thermogenic brown fat!

The researchers also show that with prolonged exposure to cold, these "cold bacteria" induce changes to the structure and function of the gut that enable more glucose to be absorbed.

In the short-term, this extra fuel can be used by the brown fat to generate heat, but in the long-term, some of these extra calories probably go towards building white fat and thus weight gain.

pubmed.ncbi.nlm.nih.gov/26638070

www.drsharma.ca/cold-exposure-promotes-gut-microbes-that-stimulate-brown-fat

Cold and Heart Rate Variability

Another study shows that cold exposure in the back of the neck does increase Heart Rate Variability, a marker of cardiac health. We want a higher HRV.

("Effects of Cold Stimulation on Cardiac-Vagal Activation in Healthy Participants: Randomized Controlled Trial". *JMIR*FormRes.2018Jul-Dec;2(2): e10257.)

www.ncbi.nlm.nih.gov/pmc/articles/PMC6334714

Cold exposure also increases growth hormone stimulation more than exercise alone. Therefore, combining cold therapy and exercise amplifies the benefits.

Another interesting study showed people who swam in ice water and its effects. The study showed a jump in the participants' glutathione levels compared to the control group. Glutathione is one of the most important antioxidants in the body. This antioxidant depletes with age and is vital, especially for phases I and II detox in the liver.

pubmed.ncbi.nlm.nih.gov/8063192

Thyroxine, a thyroid hormone, is also increased following cold exposure. This hormone plays a role in increasing our resting metabolism, allowing the body to burn more calories without any extra effort.
physoc.onlinelibrary.wiley.com/doi/pdf/10.1113/jphysiol.1974.sp010647

Great heart health, gut microbiota health, fat-burning capabilities, thyroid health, blood sugar regulation, increased glutathione levels, and heart rate variability, all with cold exposure!

Cold Throughout the Day

When it comes to working throughout the day in very cold temperatures, that's not ideal. We only want to do this process for minutes at a time. This isn't about "shivering" to get the benefits of these hormonal changes and fat deposit changes. This is about activating the hormones properly to do that work for you.

That being said, your body temperature at night, while you sleep, should be lower.

Studies have shown that you can increase your levels of brown fat from the comfort of your own bed. In one study, they showed that subjects sleeping in cooler temperatures (19 degrees C or 66 degrees F) had a 42% increase in brown fat plus a 10% increase in fat metabolic activity after just one month.

www.nih.gov/news-events/nih-research-matters/cool-temperature-alters-human-fat-metabolism

Are you ready to upgrade your health? The best way is to get some cold in your life every single day. It's usually the most intense part of Regan's day but the part that he now enjoys the most.

Your Challenge: Daily Cold Showers. Start with just 20 seconds! If you are feeling adventurous, you can try Cryotherapy, an ice bath, jumping in a cold lake, or the ocean, etc.

It's going to be a little uncomfortable, but you can do it! Do it at the beginning or end of your shower. If you have an autoimmune condition, be sure to finish with hot water after and don't end on cold. It will become easier with time.

Sing "Happy Birthday" twice, and that's about 20 seconds. If there is no one around, use expletives as much as you need. It's been shown to help.

Peptide

Sarcotropin IPA, the circulation, fat-burning, and brain-boosting peptide.

Sarcotropin IPA is a peptide, amnio acid, and vitamin blend that has been shown to increase IGF-1 levels by 16%, improve muscle mass by nearly 10%, and decrease visceral (organ) fat by 10%, all in just three months. This popular formula has made it through phase three clinical trials for Sarcopenia and is one of my favorites.

Sarcotropin IPA helps increase circulation, and is specifically designed to build muscle mass and avoid muscle atrophy. It also stimulates the brain and increases growth hormone without increasing appetite. It's a great aid in your cold exposure journey and is sure to maximize the health of your circulatory system.

Chapter Nine
Timed Eating

Reverse Aging with One Simple Rule

Mindset Number Nine
It's not just about how much I eat,
it's when I choose to eat.

Just by changing the timing of your meals, you can transform your metabolic function.

> *"Evidence is accumulating that eating in a six-hour period and fasting for 18 hours can trigger a metabolic switch from glucose-based to ketone-based energy, with increased stress resistance, increased longevity, and a decreased incidence of diseases, including cancer and obesity."*
> ~Rafael de Cabo, Ph.D. and Mark P. Mattson, Ph.D.

Timed Eating and Fat Loss

Circadian Code by Sachin Panda PhD highlights a study he did on obese mice with diabetes. He wondered if time restriction would change things in their metabolism.

Dr. Panda chose an eight-hour window for feeding. (This was actually based on the schedule of the student performing the study!) On weekdays, they did eight-hour timed eating, then on weekends, the mice could eat whenever they wanted. Another group of mice could eat 24 hours a day, every day. The same food was provided to both groups of mice with the same number of calories. He found the mice that had access to the same food as the timed eating group, but grazed all day every day (not within a timed eating window) actually became overweight mice.

After seven weeks, the mice eating in a timed window on weekdays lost almost 38% more fat than the mice who had 24/7 access to food. They also had lower levels of insulin resistance, obesity was gone, and they were stronger and healthier. These results came just from keeping the calories eaten within an eight-hour window five days a week!

Timed Eating and Metabolism

Researchers from the University of Alabama conducted a study with a small group of obese men with prediabetes. They compared a form of intermittent fasting called "early time-restricted feeding," where all meals were fit into an early eight-hour period of the day (7 am to 3 pm), or spread out over 12 hours (between 7 am and 7 pm). www.sciencedirect.com/science/article/pii/S1550413118302535

Neither group gained or lost weight, but after five weeks, the eight-hours group had dramatically lower insulin levels and significantly improved insulin sensitivity, as well as significantly lower blood pressure. The best part? The eight-hour group also had significantly decreased appetite. *They weren't starving!*

Just changing the timing of meals by eating earlier in the day and extending the overnight fast significantly benefited metabolism, even in people who didn't lose a single pound.

Another study showed how "Ten-Hour Time-Restricted Eating Reduces Weight, Blood Pressure, and Atherogenic Lipids in Patients with Metabolic Syndrome": pubmed.ncbi.nlm.nih.gov/31813824

- 10 hours of time-restricted eating (TRE) in metabolic syndrome (MetS) promotes weight loss.

- TRE in MetS reduces waist circumference, percent body fat, and visceral fat.
- TRE in MetS lowers blood pressure, atherogenic lipids, and glycated hemoglobin.
- Benefits of TRE are "add-ons" to statin and anti-hypertensive medications.

Timed Eating and Circadian Rhythm/Horary Clock

You know this now from our chapter on Sleep, but here's a refresher. A circadian rhythm, or circadian cycle, is a natural, internal process that regulates the sleep–wake cycle and repeats roughly every 24 hours. It can refer to any process that originates within an organism and responds to the environment.

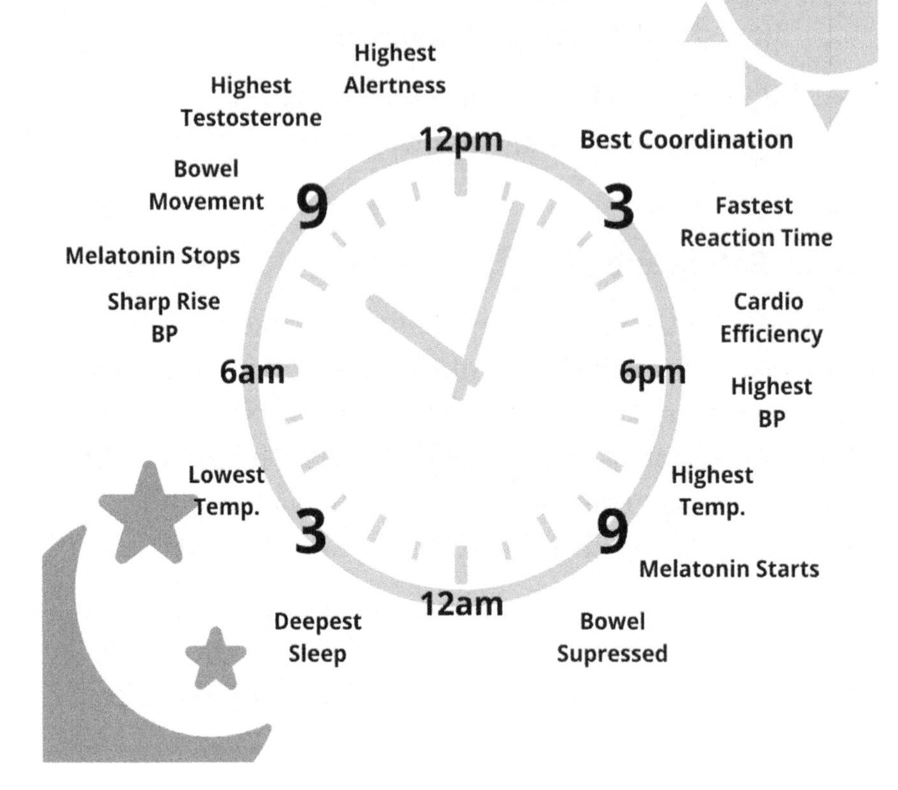
CIRCADIAN
RHYTHM
Highest
Alertness
Highest
Testosterone
12pm
Best Coordination
Bowel
Movement
9
3
Fastest
Reaction Time
Melatonin Stops
Sharp Rise
BP
Cardio
Efficiency
6am
6pm
Highest
BP
Lowest
Temp.
Highest
Temp.
3
9
Melatonin Starts
12am
Deepest
Sleep
Bowel
Supressed

The above graphic shows how important it is to stop eating well before bedtime so that your body can go through its natural processes and focus on sleep, rejuvenation, and repair. It shouldn't be focused on digesting food!

If you skipped ahead, be sure to reference back to our deep dive into Sleep Hygiene and use the above clock to your advantage.

As for the Horary cycle, it's very similar and takes these natural rhythms into account from the perspective of traditional Chinese medicine and organ health. Like seasons, we go through phases throughout the day including the elements of earth, fire, water, wood, and metal.

Check out the diagram below. Your major detox organs, hormones, and respiratory health are being rejuvenated while you sleep!

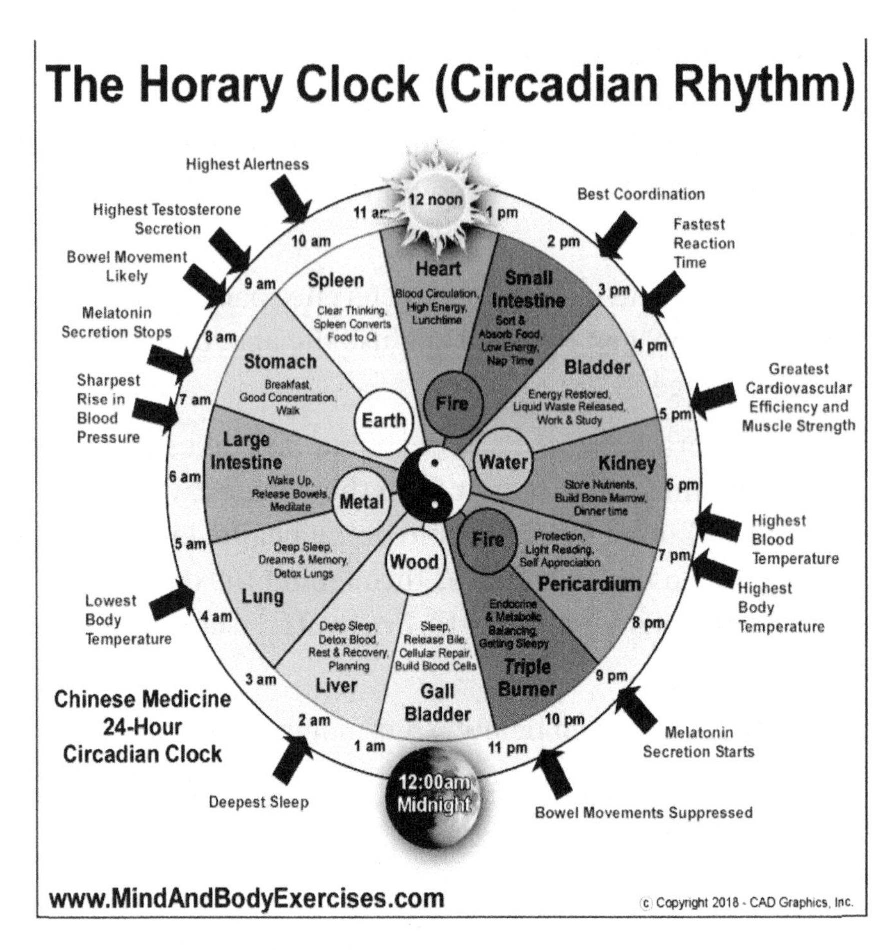

www.mindandbodyexercises.com

Having a healthy circadian rhythm where your body is aligned with nature keeps your "clock" ticking soundly!

You get to enjoy great benefits, including ease of function, such as:

- Better Release of Insulin
- Cardiovascular Strength
- Better Liver Function
- Blood Sugar Balance
- Improved Mood
- Decreased Risk of Disease
- Better Alertness and Cognitive Abilities
- Improved Sleep Quality
- Improved Metabolism

About 33% of your body has genes that are regulated by circadian rhythm!

I'd say it's well worth it to work in conjunction with the way nature intended, rather than doing the opposite and feeling the extreme negative effects of the inverse of all of the above! Brain fog, fatigue, irritability, weight gain, stress, increased risk of disease? No, thank you!

I say this and yet, many do these things all the time.

- "I'm a night owl," and they stay up past 10 pm only to sleep in very late and throw the whole process off.
- "I have to eat late."

- "My best creativity is in the middle of the night!"

Hey, I get it. You've grown used to certain patterns that are comforting, or you feel your schedule doesn't allow for this process. Think of it this way. If you are a parent (or even if you aren't, pretend you are one for a moment), what do you think would happen if you put your kids on your same routine of going to bed late, sleeping in late, and/or not getting much sleep at all? I'm sure you could guess you'd get tantrums, crying spells, anxiety, extreme fatigue, and the need to nap a lot by day, wanting to crash in front of the television instead of being outside doing fun activities in the sunshine and fresh air, eating/craving sugar, etc. That was me in high school!

Would you do that to your kids? Of course not!! By the way, shout-out to all the parents because in the beginning, before you've established that sleep pattern when they are infants or at times they are sick, have a bad dream, or snuck candy close to bedtime, I can imagine how hard that is the next day!

It's not about perfection. You simply do your best. This is about controlling what you can control, to the best of your abilities. Just like we all know the need for kids to get adequate sleep and follow routines, we need to treat ourselves with the same level of self care.

If your work requires crazy hours, just do your best to align within the framework you have. Let me give you an example.

When I was a performer, "work" technically started for me at 7pm, show time! It is very easy for performers to become night owls. You get ready, do your show for two or three hours and are famished afterwards, especially if you are a dancer. You want to go out and blow off some steam from all the energy you feel. You eat a big meal afterwards because you don't want to eat a huge meal before the show.

In order to avoid eating a big meal, staying up late, and getting a "second wind", I established a routine. During intermission, I'd eat some healthy fat like nuts around 8:30 pm, head home immediately after the show (no drinks for me most nights), and be in bed by 11:30 pm. That allowed me to cut off eating three hours before bed. (Otherwise, eating too close to bedtime gave me bad dreams and acid reflux.)

Then I could wake up comfortably eight hours later at 7:30/8am and move about my day. (By the way, performers then spend their days taking classes, working out, going to auditions for new work opportunities, or working secondary jobs, so they never really stop working.)

If you are someone who needs to wait to eat dinner after a show or a long shift at work, then yes, you're looking at a later bedtime and some great room darkening curtains with your evening wind-down routine. That's where you can still do wonderful grounding activities to remind your body what time of day it is. Try going outside for a walk in the sunshine upon waking, making sure to exercise by day at the time that works best for you, and following the clock the rest of the day as best you can.

For those who are working the "graveyard shift" that also comes with many challenges. For Regan's patients with that routine, he'll recommend still doing an eight-hour feeding window but shifting it to work within their schedule.

Lifestyle habits, above and beyond exercise, can perfectly align with this circadian rhythm. The evening is the ideal time to wind down with a paper book, dinner seated with friends and family to create connection, taking a warm bath or shower, having sex, or other stress-reducing activities. We teach our bodies through our daily choices.

Timed Eating and Your Natural Stem Cells

Studies show that fasting for 24 hours can regenerate your stem cells. ("Fasting Activates Fatty Acid Oxidation to Enhance Intestinal Stem Cell Function during Homeostasis and Aging" *Cell Stem Cell* Volume 22, Issue 5, 3 May 2018, Pages 769–778.e4.)

- Researchers fasted mice for 24 hours to study how the fasting state impacts intestinal stem cells and found that fasting augments intestinal stem cell function in both young and aged mice, by boosting fat metabolism.
- Using fats for energy preserves the health and function of intestinal stem cells.
- The ability to break down and use fats for energy is impaired in older individuals... unless they fast.

It's no wonder those who may practice fasting for religious reasons have already experienced these tremendous benefits.

Check out these photos for comparison. Intestinal stem cells from mice that fasted for 24 hours (right) produced much more substantial intestinal organoids than stem cells from mice that did not fast (left). (MIT 5/2018)

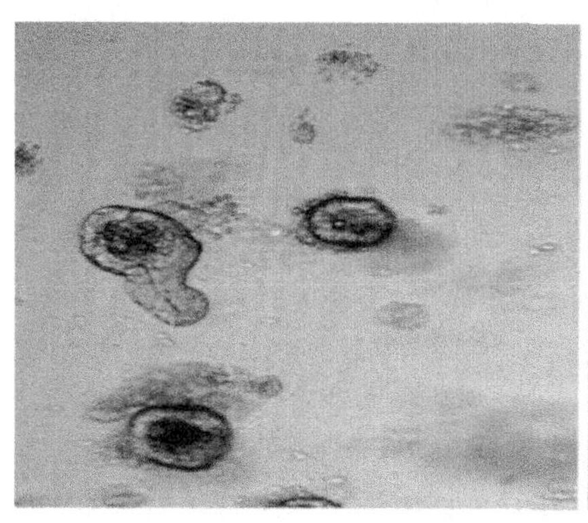
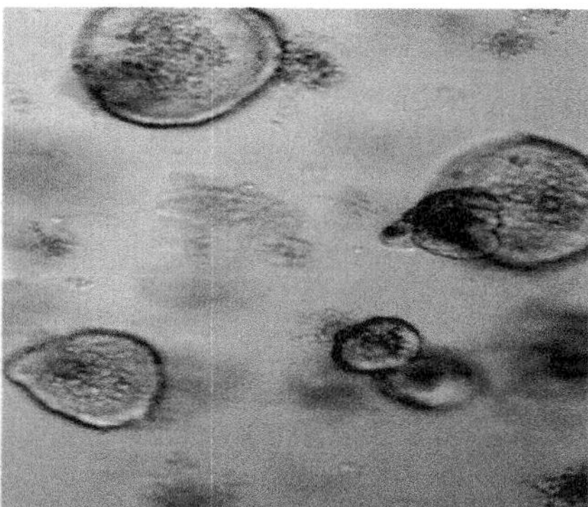

("Fasting Activates Fatty Acid Oxidation to Enhance Intestinal Stem Cell Function during Homeostasis and Aging". *Cell Stem Cell* Volume 22, Issue 5, 3 May 2018, Pages 769–778.e4.)

It was discovered that:

> *"During fasting, the intestinal stem cells in both young and old animals switch from utilizing carbohydrates to using fat as a primary energy source, and this metabolic switch is driving an improvement in stem cell function."*
> ~Omer H. Yilmaz at MIT, *Cell Stem Cell*, 2018

"Acute fasting regimens have pro-longevity and regenerative effects in diverse species, and they may represent a dietary approach to enhance aged stem cell activity in tissues."

Stem cells may function better when burning fats for fuel but lose the ability to metabolize fats efficiently as they age.

"We think we are improving the quality of the existing stem cells, rather than generating new stem cells under these conditions," Yilmaz said.

Autophagy, or the clearing out of senescent stem cells, could be contributing to this improvement.

Ketosis might be an ideal way to improve stem cell release rates.

Timed Eating and Gut Bacteria

Did you ever notice your bowel movements are better when you practice time restricted eating? Time restricted eating helps with gut motility and gut bacteria health.

Time Restricted Eating also increases a specific type of gut bacteria called Akkermansia.

"*Akkermansia muciniphila* is a mucin-degrading bacterium commonly found in the human gut. *A. muciniphila* has been inversely associated with obesity, diabetes, inflammation, and metabolic disorders. Due to its highly promising probiotic activities against obesity and diabetes, *A. muciniphila* has drawn intensive interest for research and development in recent years. A number of human and animal studies have shown that the abundance of *A. muciniphila* in the gut can be enhanced through dietary interventions."
www.ncbi.nlm.nih.gov/pmc/articles/PMC6223323

We'll talk more about this powerhouse bacteria in the Gut Optimization chapter. Just know that Timed Eating increases Akkermansia and its many benefits in the system!

The rhythms of the intestinal body clock affect metabolism, absorption of nutrients, and immunity. The intestinal body clock also communicates with the brain, the pancreas, and the liver.

Microbes living in the gut have a profound influence on the intestinal body clock, which then affects all of the other clocks. Maintaining a healthy microbiome is therefore crucial for regulating circadian rhythms.

> "In a study published in the scientific journal *Cell*, researchers analyzed fluctuations in the adherence, quantity, and metabolic activity of gut microbes in the intestines of mice every six hours for a total of forty-eight hours. They found that gut microbes have daily "routines" in which they travel to different locations throughout the intestine."
> pubmed.ncbi.nlm.nih.gov/27912059
>
> www.ascent2health.com/blog/the-link-between-gut-microbes-and-circadian-rhythms
> ~June 24, 2017 Lindsay Christensen, MS, CNS

These circadian oscillations in gut microbe activity cause the tissues of the intestine to be exposed to different microbes and their metabolites over the course of a day. The metabolites produced as a result of gut microbe circadian rhythms influence genes associated with the intestinal, pancreatic, and liver body clocks.

On the other hand, erratic eating patterns such as eating non-stop all day or eating late at night disrupts the circadian rhythms of gut microbes.

Their travels throughout the gut become disorganized, leading to disruption of the intestinal body clock and an overall uncoupling of circadian rhythms of the host in which they live (i.e., you!).

Disrupted gut circadian rhythms have been associated with insulin resistance, high cholesterol, and obesity.

Think of fasting like "correcting potholes" overnight when the cars are off in the road (no food in the system).

Should Anyone NOT do TRE?

That's a great question, and the answer is YES!

While this could go without saying, if you are someone who struggles with an eating disorder such as binge eating, bulimia, anorexia, etc., then this is not for you without the guidance of a qualified health professional (and someone who specializes in eating disorders).

If you are hypoglycemic or Type 1 Diabetic this is also not for you. Nor would it be ideal for women who are pregnant. (You are feeding two people, and you can absolutely stay in great shape while you grow your baby!)

Finally, if you still have a period and notice you need more fuel in your Luteal Phase of your cycle (that's the 10 to 14 days leading up to your period) listen to your body and do not push this. It's ideal to start this, if it's your first time, around your Follicular and Ovulatory phases which covers the first 14 days of your cycle. Day 1 is the first day you bleed, so your follicular phase starts when bleeding stops and lasts about seven to 10 days, and ovulation follows for about two to four days.

You can still fast about 12 hours easily if you stop eating three hours before bed, which is recommended whether you are fasting or not, then sleep eight or nine hours. Voilà! You just fasted 12 hours and still gave your body a break while you slept the majority of your fast! That's how I like to fast, and then depending on where I'm at in my cycle, I can gauge whether I fast 12 hours or 15 hours and break my fast at the appropriate time.

Pro Tip!

If you want something sweet after dinner or if you are still craving more food after a full meal, and you know you've eaten good quality veggies, proteins, and fats within a couple of hours, you may have Insulin Resistance.

That's where Apple Cider Vinegar can help!

Apple Cider Vinegar has been shown to have numerous benefits for blood sugar and insulin levels:

- ACV Improves insulin sensitivity during a high-carb meal by 19 to 34% and significantly lowers blood sugar and insulin responses. www.healthline.com/nutrition/15-ways-to-lower-blood-sugar
- Reduces blood sugar by 34% after eating 50 grams of white bread. (We're not saying go eat white bread and undo it with ACV, but rather, use it when you have an "oops" moment with sugar and carbs.)
- Two tablespoons of apple cider vinegar before bedtime can reduce fasting blood sugar in the morning by 4%.

- Numerous other studies in humans show that ACV can improve insulin function and lower blood sugar levels after meals.
- For these reasons, ACV can be useful for people with diabetes, pre-diabetes, or those who want to keep their blood sugar levels low for health purposes. www.healthline.com/nutrition/16-best-foods-for-diabetics.
- For flavor and additional benefits, mix with lemon or cranberry juice (unsweetened). You can even add a little stevia or monk fruit, but it tastes great with the ACV on its own! Recipe is in the Hydration chapter!

For additional benefits, check out The Smart Medicine's Energy Multiplier for blood sugar regulating ingredients including cinnamon, berberine, gymnema, and more powerhouse blood sugar stabilizers! www.thesmartmedicine.com

Challenge Time!

- No eating three hours before bed
- Minimum 12 hours off food up to 16 hours without food. Either skip breakfast if needed or eat dinner earlier. Your choice.
- Your eating window will reflect the difference in 24 hours, depending on how long you go without food, so if you're 16 hours off, choose your eight-hour

feeding window, or 15 hours off, choose your nine-hour feeding window, and so on.

- Start slow and remember, if you cut off eating three hours before bed (which we should always do) and then sleep eight hours, you have one more hour upon waking until the finish line!
- If you are a Type 1 Diabetic, hypoglycemic, have an eating disorder, or are pregnant, do not do timed eating.
- If you feel hungry during this, drink the ACV recommendations above! Water is welcome any time, and black coffee upon waking is an okay "cheat", but ideally, try and wait until you've been awake a couple of hours.
- If you start to feel shaky, you have gone too far, or you may need to address the quality of your meals during your feeding window. At that point, stop and reach out to us so we can further assist you.

Continue to eat a healthy diet in your eating window. Do not restrict. Remember, it's about reducing the window for eating, but for now, you can keep your calories the same as long as they are from good energy sources like high quality proteins, fats, and vegetables. If you don't know how much food you need, this experiment will teach you a lot. We need less than we think. If you are an athlete, as shown in the Movement chapter, you'll need more.

For more specifics on what to eat and how much, please reference the Protein, Fat, and Veggie challenge chapters!

Peptides

Epitalon: Increase Your Healthspan and Lifespan by Seven Years!

This amazing peptide resets circadian rhythms just like timed eating. Epitalon is a naturally occurring telomerase enzyme found in your pineal gland. It's expression promotes the length of the telomeres on the ends of your DNA which can result in greater stem cell activation and health.

Research done by the Epitalon pioneer, Dr. Vladimir Khavinson shows that this peptide increases longevity by seven years, decreases cholesterol, and improves cardiovascular health, amongst many other physical and mental health benefits. Some studies are finding this peptide to be very effective in cancer prevention. Khavinson, V.K., Bondarev, E., Butyugov, A.A. (2003). Epithalon peptide induces telomerase activity and telomere elongation in human somatic cells. *Bulletin of Experimental Biology and Medicine. 135*(6): 590–592

Stem Boost Protein

Mushrooms have received a lot of attention for various benefits including cellular and DNA heath. The Stem Boost formula found at thesmartmedicine.com contains Cordycepts, Reishi, Maitake, and Shitake mushrooms to enhance your body's ability to recover and heal.

Chapter Ten
Love Your Liver

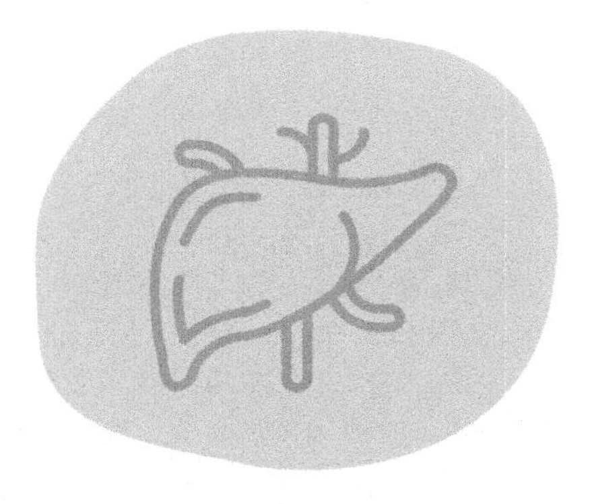

Your Hidden Healing Tool

Mindset Number Ten
By loving my liver, I allow my body to detox, heal, and support me every day.

When it comes to habit change, I wanted to give you a quick refresher on some very important things that help cultivate new habits and make them stick!

1. **Always replace an old habit that doesn't work for you with a new habit.**

   Use the structure of the old habit (the same trigger or cue) and replace the "routine", making sure it's still equally rewarding. Simply telling yourself not to do the old habit won't work. Your body has become used to a pattern and it's easier to work with the pattern in a new way!

   Ex: If you got used to eating later at night before bed, figure out what was triggering the eating. Are you truly hungry? Are you thirsty? Are you seeking comfort?

   If hungry, make it a habit of eating an earlier dinner time that is only three hours before you put your head on the pillow. Include healthy protein, fat, and veggies. Drink enough water throughout the day, and practice other routines to keep hunger at bay later at night. If it's emotional, swap out the routine of eating with something that won't derail you but still supports what you need. Cuddle up to a paperback book, drink some herbal tea, listen to some relaxing binaural beats, take a bath, etc.

2. **Use James Clear's top recommendations for habit building and make sure it's obvious, easy, attractive, and rewarding.**

   Trust me. It sticks if you do, it doesn't if you don't, and there's no shame in that. That's how it works!

Notice how any older habit (good or bad) follows this same routine.

3. **Lean on community and accountability.** Like we're doing in our live interactive HAC Community, feeling a part of something bigger works wonders. That level of support is exponentially more successful than going about this all alone. You can join our live weekly HAC community by going to www.acueastwest.com/hac.

Now let's dive into your Liver Health and WHY it's so important!

What does your liver do?

The liver is an organ located in the upper right-hand portion of the abdominal cavity, beneath the diaphragm, and on top of the stomach, right kidney, and intestines. Shaped like a cone, the liver is a dark reddish-brown organ that weighs about three pounds. It has 600 hormonal functions and 200 digestive functions. Talk about an important organ to keep healthy!

It's multifaceted and multi-talented in what it's constantly doing to support you.

- It removes potentially toxic byproducts of medications.
- It metabolizes/breaks down nutrients from foods to produce energy.
- It helps your body fight infections by removing bacteria from the blood.

- It produces most of the substances that regulate blood clotting.
- It prevents shortages of nutrients by storing vitamins, minerals, and sugar.
- It brings together amino acid chains to produce most proteins needed by the body.
- It produces bile, a compound needed to digest fat and fat soluble vitamins A, E, D and K.
- It helps regulate blood glucose.

As a reminder from the Circadian Rhythm and Horary charts we discussed, your liver is most active between 1 am and 3 am.

If you don't have a gallbladder, which helps digest and emulsify fats, you need bile salts! This should be discussed with your functional medicine practitioner alongside your PCP. Without bile production, you would have difficulty absorbing A, E, D, and K since they are fat soluble vitamins.

Ironically, the liver of other animals is one of the most nutrient dense foods you can eat! Have you ever heard of the incredible benefits of things like cod liver oil? Did your grandparents or great grandparents eat liver? They instinctively knew. Animal liver contains great raw nutrients that support your own liver.

You can soak it in goat's milk or buttermilk overnight to help take out some of the strong flavor and sauté it in onions to make it taste better!

Grab a copy of the book *Your Health Transformation* by Regan on Amazon where he talks extensively about the Liver. Check out pg. 98: "Your Liver is a Big Busy Organ". If you have liver issues, you can be grumpy, edgy, and feel irritable often, develop a potbelly, be more prone to headaches, and more prone to a lot more issues as we'll discuss below. This is why it's so important to give your liver love!

Your liver metabolizes hormones, including Estrogen!

If Estrogens don't get out of your body, it can significantly impact your mood, weight, other hormones, brain health, etc.!

That's why it's great to do a liver detox, so it can properly do its many jobs above. Regan goes into specifics for how to do a liver detox in *Your Health Transformation*. If you would like a copy, click HERE, or search for it on Amazon.

You'll recognize pulling out a lot of the trigger foods we discussed in the chapter on Sugar, and we'll mention other chemicals and toxins to be aware of in this chapter as well. Additional supportive foods for your liver are listed in *Your Health Transformation* as well as portioning your macronutrients (veggies and fats) while eliminating animal proteins temporarily.

We LOVE good quality animal proteins, as you'll learn in the Protein chapter, but it's important to pull back when detoxing the liver since protein breakdown can be hard on a liver that's not functioning optimally. Think of it as giving your liver a "break", just like we do with Timed Eating.

If you have never done a liver detox before, it's important to work with a functional medicine provider and run your labs first so you truly understand what is going on that is bogging down your liver in the first place. They can support you with easing into and out of the detox, preventing "herxheimer" flu-like symptoms or other effects from diving in too quickly without guidance.

In this chapter, we will focus on teaching you about liver health and doing one simple challenge at the end with powerhouse superfoods.

It's Not Just WHAT You Eat That Matters, It's How Much

When we consume any food or substance, the liver metabolizes it. Inflammatory signals get sent back to the liver not only when we consume inflammatory foods but also when we eat too much. This can lead to fatty liver disease.

White fat can only store so much energy, and the excess ends up in your liver, which causes it to become clogged. Now you have an excess of fat in the liver.

If your liver is preoccupied handling excess fat, sugar, and toxins, it struggles to handle the foods you are eating.

This is why it's so important to only eat until you are about 80% full!

Here are some additional Eating Hygiene tips to support your entire gastrointestinal system from beginning to end, along with liver health:

- Eat slowly, giving yourself at least 20 minutes for the body to signal you're full. (Yes, it takes that long!)
- Chew your foods thoroughly, until they are almost liquified in your mouth, before swallowing. That takes burden off your stomach from having to break down full pieces. Your saliva starts the breakdown for you!
- If you have acid reflux, you may have what is called "hypochlorhydria", a.k.a. low stomach acid. Sipping one teaspoon of apple cider vinegar mixed in water with meals can help. You need adequate stomach acid to break down foods and nutrients.
- Make sure you have optimal gut health (which we'll discuss next chapter), including enzymes, good gut bacteria from fermented foods and probiotics, and a sealed (not leaky) gut. Leaky gut is discussed extensively in the Optimize Your Gut Chapter.
- Stop eating three hours before bed. Don't lie down on a full stomach.

Eating too much and bogging down your liver over time can lead to fatty liver disease and, even worse, to NASH (NonAlcoholic SteatoHepatitis). That's when the liver gets scarred, and it's irreparable. You don't hear much about this since there's no drug for it. Big Pharma hasn't come up with any drugs for this after spending tons of money trying.

The only way to correct it is through lifestyle. Otherwise, you'd need a liver transplant if it gets out of control.

This isn't just for adults. The number one reason for kids needing a liver transplant is fatty liver disease. Get kids to eat clean, whole foods and appreciate it. Taste buds change, and what you choose to feed them has the greatest impact on their health and their ability to avoid preventable diseases.

In the United States, the prevalence of fatty liver disease ranges from 10 to 46%, and liver biopsy based studies report a prevalence of NASH at one to 17%. Systematic reviews suggest NAFLD prevalence in adults is probably 25 to 33%, while NASH prevalence is two to 5%.

NASH is the liver manifestation of a metabolic disorder, and is the most severe form of non-alcoholic fatty liver disease (NAFLD). NASH is closely related to the triple epidemic of obesity, pre-diabetes, and diabetes.

What Creates Fatty Liver?

SUGAR, for one! That's right. Be sure to review the importance of cutting out sugar outlined earlier.

Also, overconsumption of alcohol, Acetaminophen (Tylenol), or any other NSAID pain medicine that has to be metabolized by the liver can bog it down (not to mention the impact of NSAIDs on your stomach as well).

One of the Worst Myths of the Century

Healthy fats do NOT create fatty liver or contribute to a myriad of diseases as we were once taught. Healthy consumption of healthy fats is not a leading cause of obesity.

When you eat sugars like sucrose, glucose, honey, fructose, agave, maple syrup, coconut sugar, etc., they cause an insulin spike. Glucose immediately converts the fructose to triglycerides and stores them. Where?
In your liver.

If sugar is so bad for our health, and can cause FLD, obesity, diabetes, and more, why is it so commonly snuck into foods? The industries that make them know that sugar lights up your brain, tastes good, and makes you addicted. They want you to buy more.

Artificial drinks do the same thing, so don't reach for the diet soda! It confuses your blood sugar and puts the body into a stress response, breaking down more fatty acids and storing them in the liver (where you don't want it). Don't simply replace the above sugary drinks and foods with fake sweeteners. Use stevia or monk fruit for that "sweet" replacement instead, if needed. Most foods (once your taste buds adjust) taste great and sweet enough on their own!

It's important to limit even whole fruit consumption (fructose) to no more than 25g of fructose per day. A whole piece of fruit (not dried, not sugar coated, and about the size of your fist) is plenty of nature's candy. One small apple has about 12 grams of fructose, whereas grapes, mangos, bananas, and other fruits have a lot of fructose and should be eaten in moderation or taken out entirely if you struggle with blood sugar issues/diabetes/FLD. Berries are another good way to get a little sweet without the negative side effects. It's also better to eat fruits at night when you are more insulin sensitive. (Insulin sensitivity is a good thing. You don't want the opposite, which is Insulin Resistance.)

What Happens as Sugar Enters the Body?

When glucose is circulating in the blood of a healthy individual, it docks on the surface of a cell and the receptors take it into the cell to absorb as energy.

Insulin plays an important role in this process. In Type I Diabetics, there's not enough insulin being produced by the pancreas to get sugar into the cell. Whereas in Type II Diabetics, there's Insulin Resistance and glucose isn't able to find its way into the cell despite the presence of insulin. The cells reject the sugar.

High glucose is toxic to beta cells (which make insulin in your pancreas) and destroys them. This is why diabetics who just eat whatever they want and take insulin for the high glucose are getting worse. They are killing off more and more beta cells in their pancreas and needing more and more insulin support as a result, creating a vicious cycle and a breeding ground for IR!

Are we solely dependent on insulin alone to get sugar into the cell? It turns out the answer isn't what we have previously thought.

What Happens to Sugar Once in the Cell?

There are four different GLUT-type receptors that travel to the surface of your cells to take glucose from insulin into the mitochondria (the energy powerhouse of your cells).

GLUT 1 is insulin dependent, meaning it needs insulin to shuttle glucose into the blood and heart.

GLUT 2 helps with the liver, pancreas, and small intestines and is also insulin dependent. This, along with GLUT 1, requires high potassium. Potassium creates a chain that opens the door for the cell to let glucose in. Foods like avocados, olives, beet greens, and leafy greens are high in potassium to help you reach your quota. Salmon is also terrific! While bananas can be a good source, they are also very high in sugar which wouldn't be ideal to keep blood sugar in check.

GLUT 3 activates for the brain, sperm, and neurons. While it's insulin dependent, it can function with low potassium.

When those GLUT receptors ignore insulin knocking on the door, you become Insulin Resistant (IR). Even a Type I Diabetic can become insulin resistant because the beta cells in the pancreas no longer produce insulin.

The good news is there are things we can do to support this process and bypass it entirely!

As it turns out, GLUT 4 gets glucose into the skeletal muscle, adipose tissue, and heart, but ***doesn't require insulin*** or high potassium to do so **during exercise!**

For example, the more you exercise, the more the GLUT4 receptors come to the surface and take glucose in without the need for beta cells functioning and making insulin. Therefore, your body is more efficiently using up the glucose in your blood without the need for insulin when you exercise, especially with weight training. This is a win/win!

While you do need to be able to produce insulin in general, you want to be able to use as little insulin as possible to create blood sugar regulation and have insulin do its many other tasks for you. You don't want your pancreas to work hard or need to pump out a lot of insulin to keep your blood glucose in check, or you are well on your way to creating Type II Diabetes! That's a sign you are creating fatigue and dysfunction with unnecessary stress to the pancreas.

Check out this inflammatory cascade of what happens when insulin comes into play:

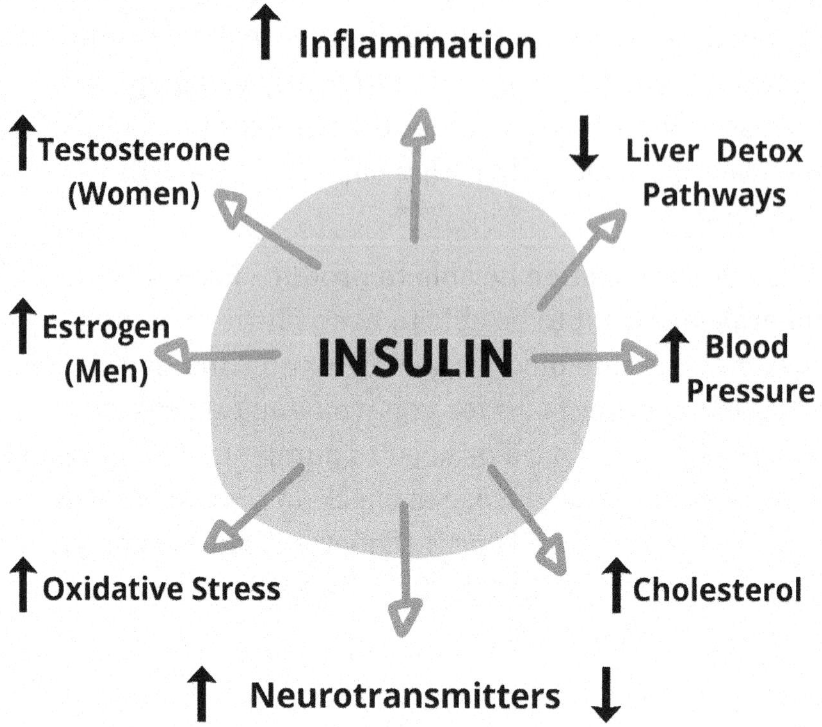

↑ Inflammation

↑ Testosterone (Women)

↓ Liver Detox Pathways

↑ Estrogen (Men)

INSULIN

↑ Blood Pressure

↑ Oxidative Stress

↑ Cholesterol

↑ Neurotransmitters ↓

As you've learned, most things inherent in the body are neither 100% bad nor 100% good. Everything works together and must be balanced to function properly.

What Else Can Be Done to Keep Insulin Levels in Check?

The more muscle you have on the body, the more your body uses up glucose 24 hours a day. The more muscle tissue you have, the more glucose you eat up even in the absence of insulin.

Do you know what happens when you have a healthy liver AND more healthy muscle mass? You prime your body to be a fat burning machine!

To prevent fatty liver disease, along with exercise, muscle gain, and not eating sugary foods or chemicals, you can also utilize the power of TRE (Time Restricted Eating).

All the sugar in the liver takes about 12 hours to burn up before it starts using up fat as an energy source. In a nutshell, TRE prompts the liver to do this process faster.

How Do You Know the Health of Your Liver?

Check your blood work!

Ideally, you want blood glucose levels to be about 75 to 90 mg/dl range when doing blood work in a fasting state. That's ideal, not the same as what conventional medicine would consider "normal" which is under 100 mg/dl. A blood glucose level of 101 to 126 mg/dl is considered pre-diabetic, and over 126 mg/dl is diabetic range.

Hemoglobin A1C takes a volume of your blood and looks at how much glucose sticks to the hemoglobin proteins in red blood cells. Those red blood cells don't recycle for 120 days, so you get a solid average for checking blood sugar levels! However, this isn't the only marker of blood sugar health or the only one you want your provider to look at. A healthy A1C should be between 4.9 and 5.5%. Pre-diabetes is about 5.7 to 6.4%, and above 6.4% is diabetic territory. This CAN be positively changed with diet, especially for Type II Diabetics and for Type I as well!

Regan and I both have checked our blood as healthy adults only to notice our HA1C had crept up to a non-ideal number. You don't have to be overweight or experiencing symptoms to have blood sugar irregularities. This is why it's important to check your labs, at bare minimum, once a year.

At that time, in my life, my results showed 5.7, so knowing I could impact it with diet and lifestyle, I made immediate changes, cut back on sugar. The next time I ran my labs, I was back down to 5.4! I've even gotten it to 5.1 being very diligent with sugar.

The sad truth is, it's been discovered that two-thirds of individuals do not achieve their target HA1C. However, we know this is achievable through diet and lifestyle. This brings us back to Regan's initial point in the beginning of the book, where he tells how many individuals answered a survey believing themselves to be healthy when, in fact, they are not by basic standards. (Saydah SH, *et al. JAMA* 2004; 291:335–342. Liebl A, *et al. Diabetologia* 2002; 45:S23–S28.)

Another important marker of liver and blood sugar health is C-peptide, which is the peptide that's attached to dormant insulin. As the body is making insulin, it reaches a "dormant state" where it attaches to C-peptide. The second the insulin becomes activated, the C-peptide is cleaved off and floats around in the bloodstream.

If you have C-peptide in your blood, that means your beta cells are working and you're making insulin.

C-Peptide should be 1 to 5, but not below 1. Sadly, more and more adults are seeing low levels of C-Peptide from autoimmune attacks on the pancreas, creating Type I Diabetes. Children and adults alike are being diagnosed with Type I Diabetes.

In a Kaiser Study, it was found that, in 3,000 people, each point above a fasted glucose of 84 mg/dl increases the risk of developing Type II Diabetes by 6% in the next nine years!

pubmed.ncbi.nlm.nih.gov/18501234

Similarly, studies have also shown that lowering Hemoglobin A1C by 1% decreases your risk of dying from diabetes by 21%, decreases microvascular complications by 37% (less likely to go blind or have kidney failure), and decreases myocardial infarction by 14%! (Stratton IM, *et al. BMJ* 2000; 321:405–412)

Some sources say that 92% of patients with diabetes had diabetic complications including diabetic neuropathy, glaucoma, cataracts, heart attacks, stroke, etc. www.ncbi.nlm.nih.gov/pmc/articles/PMC3870323

Blood work can definitely surprise many! Issues, once they have reached the surface, have already hit a much later state of imbalance. You want to catch disease within the blood work when it's veering off the ideal path before it manifests into full-blown disease, like diabetes. Blood work is such an informative way of telling us if we are on track with our diet and lifestyle or not.

Doing these habits can significantly improve your blood markers and testing across the board without first jumping to medications! These studies show you the power of getting our markers in ideal range and getting the body working for you as it's meant to.

When testing patients, Regan and his team also make sure to cover ALT, AST, Triglycerides, HDL to LDL ratio, LDL levels (which show how well you metabolize blood sugar), overall cholesterol levels, and oxidative stress to see how your liver health is doing.

Glutathione, a powerful antioxidant that supports phase II liver detoxification, can be measured with certain tests along with other antioxidants.

If you are curious to know your ongoing blood glucose levels throughout the day, you can buy over-the-counter monitors or see if your local pharmacy offers one through Good Rx for a discount! Seeing the blood glucose not just as a snapshot in time (at the time of your blood draw) but throughout the day as you eat and do different activities can be hugely informative for you and the provider you are working with.

Diabetes isn't just a problem all on its own. It can lead to other deadly diseases and issues such as blindness, kidney disease and renal failure, neuropathy, limb amputation, stroke, and a host of other unwanted conditions and comorbidities.

If you want to dive down the rabbit hole of blood sugar regulation and how vitally important it is (not just for Diabetics but for ALL of us) please check out Benjamin Bickman's book *Why We Get Sick.*

But wait, there's even more to liver health than diet and exercise.

Other Lesser Known Causes of Insulin Resistance = Toxins!

1. Outdoor Air Pollution
2. Indoor Air Pollution
3. Pesticides and Herbicides
4. Plastics (food wrap, containers, water bottles, etc.)
5. Industrial and Auto Exhaust
6. Dental Restorations
7. Factory farmed animal products (hormone injected, antibiotics)
8. Toxic cosmetic, grooming, cleaning, and body products

Let's take a closer look at Air Pollution.

A study revealed that 3.2 million new diabetes diagnoses that occurred worldwide in 2016 were caused by air pollution. That same year, air pollution caused 14% of total diabetes that occurred and 150,000 new cases in the

U.S annually. www.conserve-energy-future.com/causes-effects-solutions-of-air-pollution.php

> *In the case of diabetes, these harmful particles in the air enter the blood and obstruct insulin from converting blood glucose into energy for the well-being of the body.* ~Dr. Philip Landrigan, the dean for Global Health at Ichan School of Medicine at Mount Sinai in New York

Fun Fact: The Peptide Thymosin Alpha-1 as well as well as herbs like Astragalus and Cordyceps can be very supportive to the immune system, along with eliminating toxins when you do have control over your environment.

Even greater concern than outdoor pollution is the polluted air in your home! The many things that are sometimes invisible to the eye/scentless to the nose within your home can boggle the mind. Check out this infographic of the toxins to look out for within your home environment.

Indoor Air Pollution-#1 Contributor

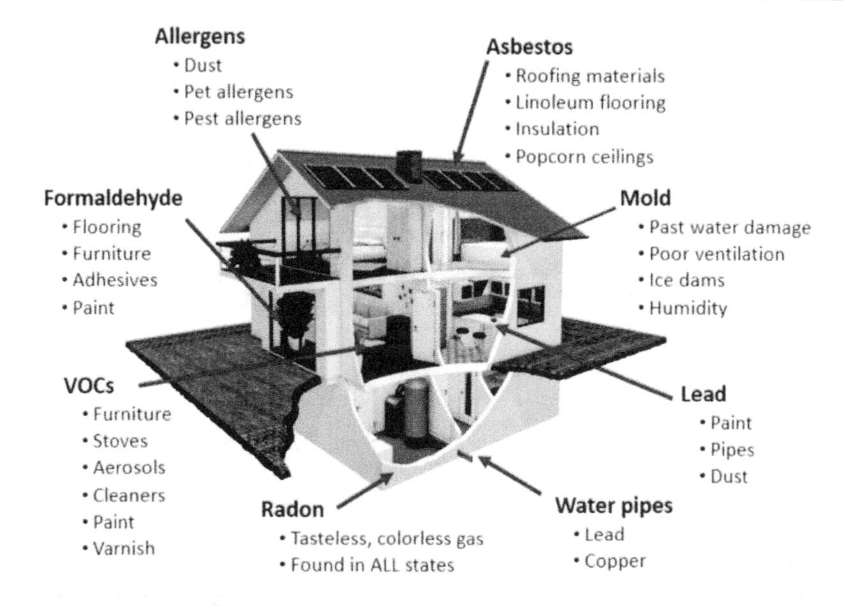

What do toxins have to do with your liver?

While the obvious stands out as bogging down the liver from functioning at its best, another interesting truth is that it causes Insulin Resistance!

Additional chemicals/toxins to watch out for by name and where they show up are below:

DIOXINS

- Produced by incineration and combustion
- Produced by the manufacture of chlorine containing products such as pesticides, wood preservatives, and the bleaching of paper

- Accumulates in human fat tissue and animals high on the food chain
- Decreases T4, T3, and testosterone. Both estrogenic and anti-estrogenic

DIOXIN CONTRIBUTORS

Paper, Pesticides, & Steel Byproducts

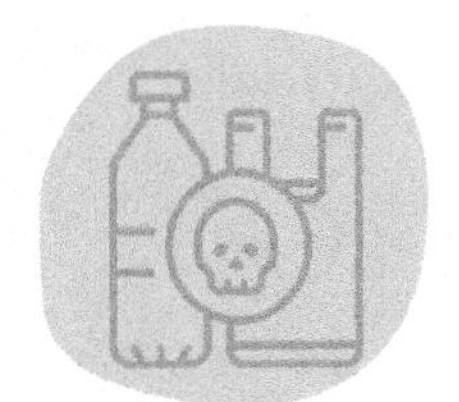

Incineration of PCVs & Plastics

Volcanic Eruptions & Forest Fires

Thermal Power Plant & Automotive Emissions

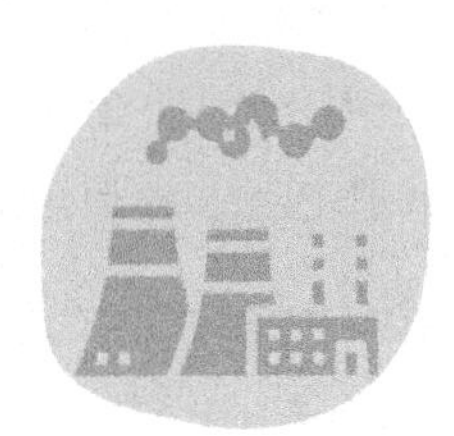

Waste Incineration

PCBs

- Used as coolant, lubricant, and insulation for electrical equipment
- In paints, plastics, dyes, and rubber
- Makes wood and plastics non-flammable
- Accumulates in human fat, the food chain, and found in rivers and lakes
- Same effects as dioxin plus low birth weight, delayed neurodevelopment, low IQ, weakened immune system, and some behave like estrogen.

BISPHENOL-A (BPA)

- A compound found in polycarbonate plastics
- Used in the manufacture of compact discs, plastic bottles, lining of metal food cans, and dental sealant
- Estrogenic influences-binds to ER+ breast cancer cells
- Decreases sperm count and increases prostate size

PHTHALATES

- Additive to PVC plastics to make them soft, flexible and strong (ex: toys)
- Carpet backing, paints, glues, insect repellents, hairspray, and nail polish

- Anti-androgenic-prenatal exposure causes hypospadias, undescended testicles
- Suppressed ovulation, estradiol production, and PCOS (rat studies)

Plastics

If you are looking for where to start cleaning up the toxins in your life, start by eliminating plastics around eating and drinking.

Plastics and the chemicals within them when ingested through water bottles, plastic storage containers for food, plastic wrap, and other plastic storage can cause what's called "molecular mimicry" like gluten and casein.

The plastics bind to estrogen receptors and continue to circulate through the body (not eliminated) where they get deposited into fat cells. The body is seeking to protect you from a toxin dump by keeping it locked up within the fat cells.

Plastics can decrease sperm count in men, increase prostate size, can cause breast cancer, uterine cancer, and other issues.

The faster you can slowly wean off plastics in your life, one at a time, the better. This was a challenge for our Thyroid HAC, and while we don't expect people to get rid of all plastics within one week, now's the time to start weaning off little by little!

Exercise: Nature's Medicine for Insulin Resistance

A large government-funded clinical trial known as the Diabetes Prevention Program found that the combination of diet improvements and 150 minutes of weekly exercise were roughly twice as effective as metformin at preventing the development of Type 2 diabetes among people at high risk for the disease. www.niddk.nih.gov/about-niddk/research-areas/diabetes/diabetes-prevention-program-dpp

"Physical activity creates muscle contractions, which allows the muscles to take up blood glucose directly without the need for insulin," says Sheri Colberg-Ochs, first author of the position statement and a professor emerita of exercise science at Old Dominion University. "Exercise is like a separate dose of insulin that always works," she adds.

During the period of eating after exercise, the food you consume will be used in a couple of ways: converted to glycogen and stored in your muscles or burned as energy immediately to help with the recovery process, with minimal amounts stored as fat.

Takeaway: Exercise every day and ideally before meals. Walk after you eat dinner! Loving your liver with exercise is yet another benefit of the many we shared in the Movement chapter.

Above and beyond exercise, if you are needing additional support for IR, Berberine, Gymnema, Cinnamon, and other supplements can be very beneficial for blood sugar regulation. More and more studies are coming out on their impact being just as powerful, if not moreso, compared to certain medications.

We offer this in a supplement called Energy Multiplier if you want to check that out at www.thesmartmedicine.com.

Three Things to Eat for Liver Health

Three very powerful foods we want you to eat for your liver health, and which are a part of this week's challenge are...

1. Garlic
2. Turmeric
3. Beets

Garlic

Garlic is found in the alliums family of food. It's a sulphur rich food that helps metabolize components that the liver usually handles.

Vitamin B in garlic lowers homocysteine in the liver which lowers inflammation and helps move the liver along in its detox.

If garlic hurts your stomach, try cooking it! It's very powerful (antimicrobial) by nature, so it can kill things off.

Garlic is delicious and a perfect add-on to most savory dishes.

Turmeric

Turmeric tells the liver cells to become more receptive to LDL (Low Density Lipoprotein).

ALT is the fatty liver marker.

In a study with 60 participants with high ALT liver enzymes, 30 took turmeric for 12 weeks and had lower levels of ALT and other liver markers compared to 30 in the placebo group, which stayed the same. pubmed.ncbi.nlm.nih.gov/30653773

You can have a lot of fun with turmeric. Turmeric can be thrown in a latte to make "golden milk", used with rice or veggie dishes (it creates an amazing orange color), meat stir fry, and more!

You can also take it as a supplement in concentrated form. You'll want to take curcumin (a component of turmeric) for its powerful anti-inflammatory benefits.

Beets

Beets love your liver! They contain pectin which is a fiber that helps the liver dump its toxins by binding to them and clearing them out!

Betaine activates your digestive system and contributes to the natural detoxification process, helping all phases of detox.

Betaine breaks down proteins to support your body with extracting the amino acids. It also increases the production of glutathione!

There are different kinds of beets: baby beets, golden beets, red beets that help build up your blood, etc. Don't forget to also eat the beet greens!

Fun fact: Beet greens are the most heavily dense supply of potassium! In case you were wondering, you can eat pickled beets as well.

Finally, beets will pump up your nitric oxide levels, which can positively impact blood pressure, heart health, and performance during exercise.

Your Challenge: For the next week, grab these three bad boys at your local health food store and look up some fun ways to incorporate them into your meals! Add at least one of these to your diet every day.

Tip: When eating beets, if you are buying them raw, be sure to cook them, and then, like rice or potatoes, store them in the fridge and cool them before you eat them. Since they are naturally a bit higher in sugar, this helps offset that effect. Eat them whole and not juiced!

Peptide

Tesamorelin for Liver Health

Tesamorelin is a 44-chained amino acid that has been studied extensively in diminishing belly fat and restoring normal liver enzyme production. This peptide has been incredibly helpful with my patients who have struggled to give up excessive alcohol consumption. They've remarked that they just don't like alcohol after using Tesamorelin, and they also see a decline in belly fat and an improvement in cognitive function.

This peptide keeps your hypothalamus and pituitary turning out hormonal signals necessary for optimal health. It also signals your liver to metabolize those hormones, so it can move on with aiding your body in digestion and detoxification.

Chapter Eleven
Optimize Your Gut

OPTIMIZE
YOUR GUT

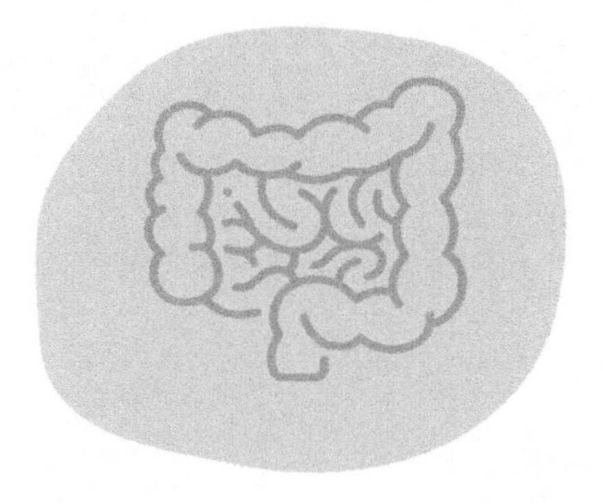

Your Second Brain

Mindset Number Eleven
I choose to give my gut exactly what it needs because my entire health depends on it.

Step 1 to Optimal Gut Health: Identify Your Triggers

Do you have certain triggers when it comes to food? Whether it's brought on by physical or mental/emotional circumstances, or just seeing/smelling/tasting the food itself, what are those "trigger foods" you gravitate towards, and what is the environment in which it tends to come up? Write them all down.

A trigger can be brought on by many different internal and external factors:

- **Feelings.** We might eat more when we're stressed, lonely, or bored. Food fills the void.
- **Time of day.** We always have a cookie at 11am, or a soda at 3pm. It's just part of our routine.
- **Social settings.** Hey, everyone else is having beer and chicken wings, so we might as well join the happy hour!
- **Place.** For some reason, a dark movie theater or our parents' kitchen might make us want to munch.
- **Thought pattern.** Thinking "I deserve this" or "Life is too hard to chew kale" might steer us toward the drive-thru window.

When you find yourself eating when you're not physically hungry, or when you know that food isn't particularly nourishing, increase your awareness of your triggers by asking yourself the following questions:

- *What am I feeling?*
- *What time is it?*

- *Who am I with?*
- *Where am I?*
- *What thoughts am I having?*

Remember the food/mood journal from the beginning of the book? Even if you haven't started, now's the perfect time! Keep a log and look for patterns. This is an extremely beneficial exercise to unlock unconscious patterns and begin to reframe and develop newer habits with a lot more ease! Once you've discovered the trigger, it's far easier to approach with potential new habits that satisfy.

Swap Your Triggers with these Great Habits!

One of the biggest triggers for people when reaching for food is stress. Food can be comforting, and when we don't want to feel uncomfortable emotions, it can feel like a pleasant distraction. (Make sure you read the chapter on Stress where we discussed the full cascade effect when stress occurs in the body.)

Food isn't the only go-to for stress relief. The least effective stress relievers include: gambling, shopping, smoking, eating, drinking, playing video games, surfing the internet, and watching TV/movies for more than two hours. You do the activity and may feel good in the moment, but it doesn't resolve the emotions or circumstances, and you end up right where you started once it's done. These are avoidance techniques rather than stress-relieving tools.

These habits form when dopamine gives us a "hit" of pleasure. Dopamine feels rewarding immediately, but because it's an excitatory neurotransmitter, it actually stimulates adrenaline and initiates the stress response. (It's ironic how these activities end up leading to more stress in the short and long run when stress is what we are seeking to avoid in the first place.)

According to the American Psychological Association, the most effective stress relievers are:

- Exercising/playing sports
- Reading
- Listening to music (or try free Binaural Beats!)
- Praying/attending a religious service
- Spending time with friends and family
- Getting a massage
- Walking outside
- Meditation
- Yoga
- Engaging in a creative hobby

What are some activities that may not be on the list that you love to do, and that would support you the next time you have a trigger moment?

As mentioned in the chapter on Stress, if you would like to learn the practice of Emotional Freedom Tapping, it's designed to release emotional triggers and significantly lessen their impact on behavioral choices, especially with regard to emotional eating. You can search and find short video tutorials on how to do EFT online. There are even apps and instructors for guided practice.

Regan's favorite stress-busting tools include exercise and cold plunge.

Anne loves many activities for stress relief, and doing them even when not in a "stressed state" in order to prevent potential triggers from manifesting. They include meditation, EFT, being outside, sleep/naps, and creativity. Writing in a journal each morning, reading, listening to Binaural Beats, and using Apollo Neuro are also very enjoyable practices to get into parasympathetic mode.

When it comes to avoiding physical and emotional cravings, all of these challenges and tools you are learning will help tremendously, but we also want to make you aware of certain foods/food groups that, in and of themselves, are triggers that make the body want more. They too cause unnecessary stress on the body, and sadly, they are built to be addicting.

Processed Foods

Processed foods are scientifically engineered to be consumed in large quantities. If you can't stop, the chips are doing their job!

Junk food is designed to make us respond with compulsive, manic, gotta-have-more snack sessions. Sometimes we even mistakenly assume we are eating a healthy snack option (due to misleading marketing) when, in fact, we are not. Snacking mindlessly is even worse, as we aren't even paying attention to whether we are full or the sensation that we are eating!

If you've felt this, you're not alone (and you're not broken).

Processed foods are made not with your health in mind, but with sales in mind. Think about how there are teams devoted to making sure manufacturers of products like cereal, chips, crackers, cookies, etc. have new and interesting flavors on the horizon, fine-tune their current flavor profile, texture, color, branding, etc. to be as tantalizing to the senses as possible.

The result? Sales of processed food go up, along with our waistlines, obesity rates, the diabetes epidemic, heart disease, you name it. McDonald's is a perfect example of this. Watch the documentary *SuperSize Me* and you'll know what we mean.

This is especially harmful to kids. We are, quite literally, making our children and future generations overweight, sick, and increasing their risk of disease or furthering disease like childhood diabetes. This is serious.

If you prefer an "Eat this, Not that" depiction of what processed foods are compared to eating real whole foods, check this out:

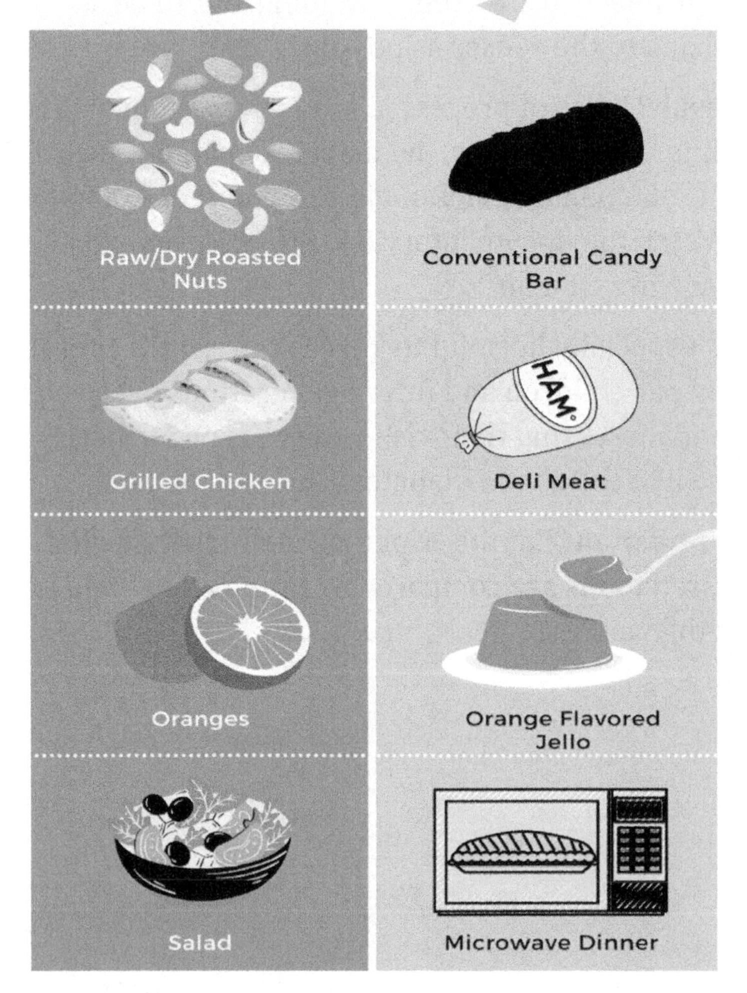
REAL FOOD
VERSUS
PROCESSED FOOD
EAT THIS, NOT THAT
Raw/Dry Roasted Nuts
Conventional Candy Bar
Grilled Chicken
HAM
Deli Meat
Oranges
Orange Flavored Jello
Salad
Microwave Dinner

Basically, if it has a laundry list of ingredients, especially things you don't recognize or can't pronounce, it's processed. Things on the outer rim of the grocery store like fruits and vegetables, meat, fish, eggs, etc. are whole foods that don't have an ingredient list.

What about Corn?

Boiled and eaten off the cob, it's pale yellow, kind of fibrous, but chewy and delicious.

Corn that's a bit processed (ground into a meal and shaped into a flat disk) turns into a soft corn tortilla. A tortilla has nice flavor and texture that makes it easy to eat and digest.

What if the corn is ultra-processed? You've removed all the fiber, isolated the starch, and then use that starch to make little triangle-shaped chips, which are fried and dusted with sweet and salty barbecue powder. Hungry yet?

That corn on the cob is yummy, but those corn-derived chips? They're... well, they're gone because someone ate them all.

Pick up most boxed/bagged processed items at the grocery store and nine times out of 10, you will see some corn derivative in the ingredients list. Next time you go to the store, I recommend you read ingredient lists as an experiment and report back how many times you saw corn listed. You can thank government subsidizing of corn crops for making it so cheap, easily accessible, and widely overused alongside crops like soy, wheat, and other grains you'll see in most processed foods.

The Scoop on Grains

Grains are processed into a slurry and pass through a machine called an extruder. With the help of high heat and pressure, whole, raw grains get transformed into airy, crispy, easy-to-digest items like cereals, crackers, cookies, etc.

In addition to changing texture and digestibility, the extrusion process also destroys certain nutrients and enzymes, denatures proteins, and changes the starch composition of a grain. This lowers the nutritional value and increases the glycemic index of the product.

What Are Emulsifiers?

Used in food to improve the "mouth feel" of a product, emulsifiers smooth out and thicken texture, creating a rich, luxurious feel.

Although there are natural emulsifiers, like egg yolk, the food industry often uses chemical emulsifiers like Polysorbate-80, sodium phosphate, and carboxymethylcellulose.

Emulsifiers are common components of processed foods consumed as part of a Western diet.

Mouse model and human intestinal tissue studies have all suggested that very low concentrations of the food emulsifier polysorbate-80 may cause bacterial

translocation across the intestinal epithelium, intestinal inflammation, and metabolic syndrome.
www.ncbi.nlm.nih.gov/pmc/articles/PMC4910713/

www.ncbi.nlm.nih.gov/pmc/articles/PMC6899614

This raises the possibility that dietary emulsifiers might be factors in conditions such as coronary artery disease, type 2 diabetes and Crohn's disease. (*NutritionBulletin* 44(4):329–349, December 2019.)

Flavor and Color Additives

Flavor additives like artificial flavoring agents or monosodium glutamate (MSG) allow food manufacturers to amplify taste without adding whole-food ingredients like fruits, vegetables, or spices. This is useful because artificial flavoring agents are cheap and won't change a product's texture. (We shared with you how many different names there are for MSG, sugar, and artificial sweeteners in the Sugar chapter.)

Coloring agents, like Yellow #5 (tartrazine) and Red #40 (allura red), are added purely for the look of food. They don't add nutrition but can increase addiction and cancer.

Recently, many large food corporations have been switching to natural food dyes, like beet powder or turmeric, to color their food products after some correlations emerged linking artificial coloring agents to behavioral problems in children.
www.webmd.com/add-adhd/childhood-adhd/food-dye-adhd

Food Additives

Human gut microbes are susceptible to antimicrobial food additives *in vitro*.

> *"Our data show that some human gut microbes are highly susceptible to antimicrobial food additives. We speculate that permanent exposure of human gut microbiota to even low levels of additives may modify the composition and function of gut microbiota and thus influence the host's immune system."*
> ~*Folia Microbiologica*, Vol. 64, pp. 497–508(2019)

The effect of additive-modified gut microbiota on the human immune system could explain, at least in part, the increasing incidence of allergies and autoimmune diseases.

> *"Changes in intestinal tight junction permeability associated with industrial food additives explain the rising incidence of autoimmune disease."*
> ~*Autoimmunity Reviews*, Vol. 14:Issue 6, pp. 479-489, June 2015.

Glucose, salt, emulsifiers, organic solvents, gluten, microbial transglutaminase, and nanoparticles are extensively and increasingly used by the food industry, claim the manufacturers, "to improve the qualities of food".
www.sciencedirect.com/topics/medicine-and-dentistry/emulsifying-agent

However, all of the aforementioned additives increase intestinal permeability by breaching the integrity of tight junction paracellular transfer.

Research shows these food additives producing leaky gut, causing dysbiosis, and changing the environment of our bacterial health could be the reason for such an increase in autoimmune conditions. We call these autoimmunogenic additives. More research is needed, but if you have autoimmunity, please avoid this.

Additional research on Dysbiosis as an Automimmune trigger:
www.ncbi.nlm.nih.gov/pmc/articles/PMC4742538

("Impact of food additives on the gut-brain axis" *Physiology & Behavior*. Vol. 192, pp. 173–176, 1 August 2018.)

- An altered microbiota can become detrimental and lead to inflammation, metabolic disorders, and even altered behavior/neuroinflammation.
- While there are many factors involved in regulating the intestinal microbiota composition, new research is showing that the pro-inflammatory signals not only impact the gut lining, but also behavior.

Food additives affect the gut-brain axis. The gut-brain axis is the two-way pathway between the digestive system and the brain. It has a huge effect on overall mood and mental well-being.

Are you wondering why conditions like ADHD, ADD, anxiety, and depression are on the rise, especially in kids? Look at the diet! The gut is now seen as your "second brain", and more and more, potentially, the first brain considering how impactful it is on disease processes.

Many functional medicine providers are finding so many patient diseases start with poor gut function, even if they seem "unrelated" on the surface.

The High Cost of Cheaper, Poor Food Choices

As a health coach, one of the biggest arguments I've received from clients not wanting to eat healthy/shop healthy is, "It's so expensive!" I get it. Organic is more expensive than conventional. Health food products that are gluten free, keto, NSF certified, non-GMO, and other labels (especially for animal protein) are more expensive than factory farmed foods, processed junk foods, and for most things that aren't good for us. Isn't that backwards? It makes me mad, and I hope it makes you mad, too!

It should be the other way around. If our government and public health institutions truly cared about our health, it would be, but it's not that way. Our food supply is created not to feed and sustain health, but to boost profits.

We have to be our own best food advocates. We have to educate ourselves and learn how to read labels (which you are doing right now!) and educate our children and future generations how to eat healthy.

We have to start moving the needle in the right direction so that, eventually, there is such high demand for healthy foods and low purchase of processed junk that manufacturers, marketers, and corporations can't help but take notice and change with consumer desire.

That's the power you have as a buyer. They make what you buy more of. They will take advantage of "fad diets", food crazes, and misleading labels knowing full well most people don't even know what they mean. It just "sounds like it's good for you."

We are giving you the tools and knowledge you need so that you are never taken advantage of by food corporations, and so you have health independence for life.

I hate to say this, but if we keep buying the junk foods just because they are cheap and taste good, despite knowing they aren't supporting us, we are fully to blame for our increased risk of weight gain, diabetes, and other health conditions.

Nothing changes unless we each make the change for ourselves and demand better. Others can care about your health, but they are not the ones making your food choices day in and day out (unless they are parents of very young kids, in which case: Parents, you can significantly influence your children's future with what you put on their plates today!).

Equipped with this information, it's meant to put you in a mindset of empowerment because you get to choose. The choices you make now are an investment into your highest good and highest long-term yield, or into you feeling worse over time. One-percent gains add up exponentially just as 1% poor choices add up every day. By choosing to be 1% better and choosing good-quality foods now, you offset the potential need in the future for expensive/harmful medications and side effects, crazy high medical bills/premiums, and potential surgeries.

If you want high energy, great libido, the ability to sustain a healthy pregnancy, the desire to look good in clothing, or really anything in life, choosing what is most important to you and your health will influence your ability to accomplish it 100%. Keep eating the cheap junk foods and you will turn on inflammatory processes and genetic predispositions that otherwise may never have occurred.

Don't let your health get out of your hands and wake up one day wondering how you got so far away from being as healthy as you want to be. No excuse is worth sacrificing your health for.

Are you fired up yet? Anger and frustration is phenomenal motivation when used wisely. Let's keep learning!

Dysbiosis or Leaky Gut: The Hidden Inflammatory Agent

Have you heard of Leaky Gut?

If you have brittle finger nails, white dots on your fingernails, skin irritation, feel tired after you eat, gas, bloating, cramping, and/or pain after eating, constipation and/or diarrhea, there's a good chance you have a leaky gut.

Leaky gut occurs when the tight junctions in the cell walls of your intestinal lining (only about a cell thick) become permeable and allows food particles to enter into the bloodstream where they don't belong.

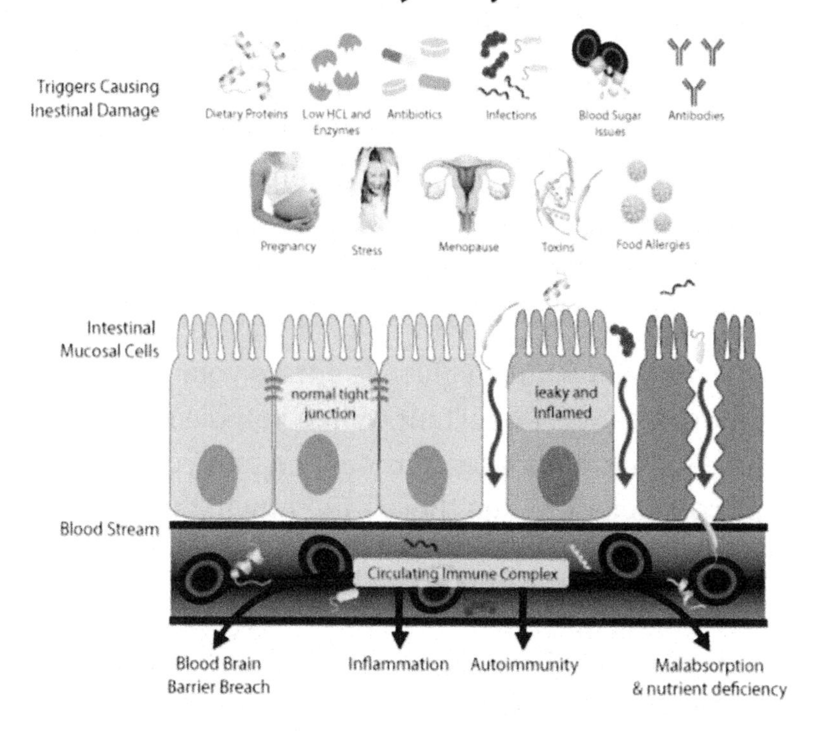

Leaky gut can make your blood more acidic, increases inflammation, can increase food sensitivities, skin conditions, brain fog, fatigue, and could be the cause for not feeling satiated after meals. It's grown a lot more common, especially with higher prevalence of processed food consumption.

What do you do to support gut lining and prevent leaky gut?

- *Akkermansia muciniphila* (Remember this?). This bacterium munches on the mucus that covers your gut lining, which encourages the intestinal barrier to produce more. This makes it stronger and thicker, preventing unwanted metabolites and toxins from entering the body that would trigger an immune response and inflammation.

- This bacterium is more abundant in lean people and less abundant in patients with obesity. Studies indicate that *Akkermansia* can help the body control sugar and fat metabolism, both of which are an issue in overweight and obesity. www.ncbi.nlm.nih.gov/pmc/articles/PMC7046546
- Managing how much glucose enters your bloodstream is important. When you have healthy levels, your body uses it as energy, and you don't put on weight. When there's too much, though, insulin tells the cells to store all the extra in your fat cells, usually around the waist.
- *Akkermansia* also produces acetate, a short-chain fatty acid that helps regulate body fat stores and appetite.

Foods that feed *Akkermansia* include:

- Pectin in apple peels (Eat the peels alone!)
- Garlic
- Cranberries
- Black tea
- Fish oil
- Bamboo shoots
- Flaxseeds
- Rhubarb extract

Additionally, the following can also prime a healthy gut:

Butyrate!

- Your bacteria love this prebiotic.
- Butyrate possesses anti-inflammatory and anti-cancer functions for your gut.
- Butyrate defends your cells from harmful substances to keep your gut healthy and disease-free.
- Butyrate is the main energy source for colonocytes, the cells which make up your gut lining.

What foods contain Butyrate?

- Grass-fed butter
- Fibrous vegetables
- Fiber, including:
    - Inulin rich foods (jerusalem artichoke, leaks, shallots and red onions, chicory root)
    - Pectin-soluble fiber (apples, plums, pulp of citrus fruits)

Resistant Starch

If you'd like to add something potentially new to your resistant starch regimen, try overnight cold gluten free rolled oats. Put the oats into a mason jar or other suitable glass container and cover with non-dairy milk (not soy) or plain water. Refrigerate overnight. Add collagen and cinnamon in the morning, if you like.

Additional examples include...

- Cooled Potatoes
  - Potatoes contain resistant starches when cooked, then cooled.
- Cooled Rice
  - Rice, when cooled for at least 24 hours, causes starch retrogradation.
- Underripe Bananas and Plantain Flour
  - When choosing bananas, go for the green. They may be tough to eat, but they are higher in resistant starch. Plantains are more resistant to digestion so trying plantain flour may help increase levels of Butyrate.

Allowing starchy foods to cool before eating them decreases the number of calories we can extract from them again. (This is mostly due to the formation of resistant starches.)

Additional Support for Healing Leaky Gut

Glutamine

Glutamine is a major nutrient to maintain intestinal barrier function in animals and humans. Depletion of glutamine results in villous atrophy, decreased expression of tight junction proteins and increased intestinal permeability. Moreover, glutamine supplementation can improve gut barrier function in several experimental conditions.

Bone Broth

Simmering bones, cartilages, and joints of chicken, beef, pork, and even fish, among others, for hours or days can provide you with digestive benefits. Bone broth is a rich source of collagen. This is the protein that helps maintain the structure and strength of connective tissues, such as those in the gut. It also contains glutamine.

When it comes to how much bone broth to drink for leaky gut, aim for two cups a day. You can also add it to your soups and smoothies.

Fermented Foods

Fermented foods such as kefir, kimchi, and sauerkraut are excellent sources for probiotics. These are beneficial microorganisms your gut needs to improve the balance of gut flora.

This will then reduce the permeability of the intestinal walls. You can also complement your fermented foods with supplements like probiotics, which contain both good bacteria and fungi.

Prebiotics are essential for bacterial health and can be found primarily in fiber-rich foods like vegetables, ginger, and turmeric.

Pea Protein

Pea protein is great for individuals with autoimmunity as well as vegans. This protein is also one of the best foods for improving the microbiome according to this study.

> "The glycated pea proteins affected the growth of gut commensal bacteria, particularly lactobacilli and bifidobacteria, whose levels increased significantly. There was a corresponding shift in the bacterial metabolites with increased levels of the short chain fatty acids (SCFAs); acetate, propionate lactate and butyrate."
> ~"Study on the impact of glycated pea proteins on human intestinal bacteria". *Int J Food Microbiol.* 2011 jan 31;145(1):267–72.

Omega-3 Fatty Acids

You can also manage a leaky gut when eating foods rich in omega-3 fatty acids like fish, seaweed, nuts, and seeds. Omega-3 assists in reducing inflammation, which is often the reason for the leaky gut symptoms.

A 2016 case study reported how these essential fatty acids change the composition of gut flora. To be specific, it promotes the growth of bacteria that produce butyrate, the short-chain fatty acid known to help improve the intestinal barrier function.

CBD

There's now research to support that CBD does indeed have a direct effect on our metabolism. In a 2016 study, researchers carefully monitored CBD and its effects on immature fat cells (preadipocytes). They surprisingly found that the cannabinoid had three ways of effecting "fat browning".

Not only did they discover how CBD played a role in the breakdown of fat, but also how it can boost the number and activity of mitochondria (increasing the body's power to burn calories) as well as reducing the production of proteins involved in creating new fat cells within the body.

["Cannabidiol promotes browning in 3T3-L1 adipocytes", *Molecular and Cellular Biochemistry*, vol. 416, pp. 131–139 (2016)]

Your Silent Metabolic Partner

The "health tax" is the toll you pay for eating low-nutrient, highly processed foods. If you eat them consistently over time, eventually, you'll pay the price with your health.

When companies use cheap, poor quality ingredients, they can sell bigger quantities without raising the price. Some people have larger populations of *Bacteroidetes* (a species of bacteria), which are better at extracting calories from tough plant cell walls than other bacteria species.

Here's an interesting example of this whole process at work. Recently, USDA researchers asked test subjects to consume 45 grams (about 1.5 servings) of walnuts daily for three weeks.

They found that, on average, people only absorbed 146 of the 185 calories in the nuts. That's 79% of the calorie content on the label.

In similar research, people also absorbed only 80% of the calories in almonds, and 95% of the calories in pistachios.

Beyond the average, there are individual differences. Some people absorb more of the energy in the nuts, while some absorb less (likely due to differing populations of bacteria in their large intestines).

What does Gut Diversity do for the body?

Say you are a meat eater, and your protein levels aren't ideal. Your iron levels are off, and you feel symptoms like gas, bloat, acid reflux, etc. There's more than just the food you are putting in your mouth at play.

What could be going on, functionally speaking, in the example above is that the gastrointestinal system isn't functioning optimally to be able to break down the protein and use it for fuel. It's getting stopped up and putrefied in the gut. This can lead to issues like SIBO and other overgrowths when not addressed.

You get energy in food from absorption in your mouth, stomach, and small intestine, but then the bacteria in your gut have their own calorie consumption and energy storage as well.

What can cause protein breakdown issues and malabsorption within the gut in the first place that leads to the above issues (which can ultimately impact your ability to accomplish your challenge in the Protein chapter as well)? (This is why we put this one first.)

- **Diversity:** There should be a wide variety of bacteria in the gut. This allows them to perform complementary activities, deter pathogens, and take over a specific job if something happens to one species. *Low diversity is a sign of dysbiosis.*

- **Balance:** Having balanced proportions of different microbes indicates that they are living in harmony. When there are too many of some or not enough of others, it's a sign that something isn't quite right. *Overgrowth and/or a lack of specific bacteria are linked to dysbiosis.*
- **Dietary fiber:** Many types of dietary fiber have a prebiotic role for the gut microbiome. Prebiotics are simply dietary fibers (and some other complex carbohydrates) that nourish beneficial bacteria in the gut. *If the diet doesn't have enough different fibers or the microbiome doesn't contain the right bacteria to break them down, this can be a sign of dysbiosis.*
- **Disease protection:** There are patterns of dysbiosis associated with common diseases. The fewer features your gut microbiome has in common with each pattern, the better your protection from illness. *Sharing several microbiome traits with a pattern linked to illness may indicate dysbiosis.*
- **Probiotics and beneficial bacteria:** These bacteria perform essential roles for human health. They promote stability and deter pathogens. That is why a healthy microbiome is, in part, defined by their presence and abundance in the gut. *Lack of beneficial and probiotic bacteria may indicate dysbiosis.*

The above is showing you why it's so important to not eat a ton of animal protein without supporting your gut microbiome first!

Why You Should Cook Your Foods

We often absorb more energy from foods that are cooked (and/or chopped, soaked, blended) because those processes break down plant and animal cells, increasing their bioavailability.

When eating raw starchy foods, we absorb very few of the calories. After cooking, however, the starches are much more available to us, tripling the number of calories absorbed.

Your Challenge! (If doing all the suggestions below feels like too much, start with just noting your triggers and slowly "crowding them out" with better options instead. Pick your biggest trigger food to start! Then add in the rest, one by one, to support gut health.)

1. **Emotional Eating Check-In:** Write down all your triggers and keep a "food/mood" journal.
2. **Remove Items** that contribute to Leaky Gut.
3. **Add In**
    a. Bone Broth
    b. Omega-3 Fatty Acids
    c. CBD
    d. Fermented Foods Daily

Chapter Twelve
Veggies

VEGGIES

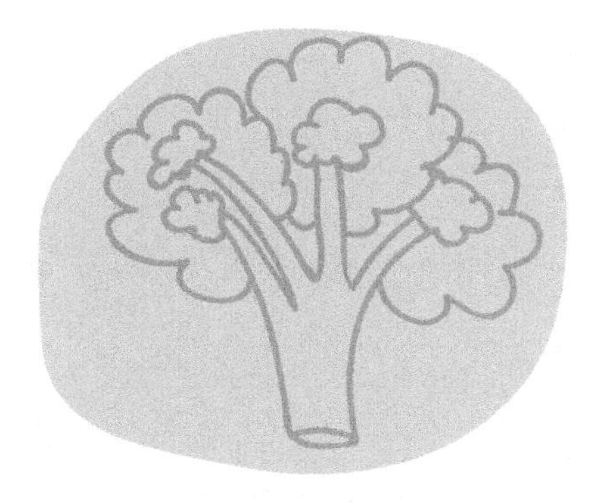

Some Things Never Change. Eat Your Veggies!

Mindset Reset
Vegetables taste delicious, and when I explore the many varieties, cook them properly, I can sense my taste buds craving them.

How to Prime Your Genetics

Genetics? But I thought this was about vegetables...

We'll get there. This is the setup to help you understand how amazingly healing vegetables really are. First, let's go over some definitions as you may have heard these terms before, but it's important to learn what they actually are and what they do.

Polyphenols: Polyphenols are a large family of naturally occurring micronutrients found abundantly in plants. There are more than 8,000 types of Polyphenols including flavonoids, tannic acid, and ellagitannin.

Antioxidants: Antioxidants are compounds that inhibit oxidation, a chemical reaction that can produce free radicals and chain reactions that may damage the cells of organisms. Antioxidants are substances that may protect your cells against free radicals, which may play a role in heart disease, cancer, and other diseases. Free radicals are molecules produced when your body breaks down food or when you're exposed to tobacco, smoke, or radiation.

Sirtuins: A family of signaling proteins involved in metabolic regulation. They are ancient in animal evolution. It is believed that sirtuins play a key role during cell response to a variety of stresses, such as oxidative or genotoxic stress, and are crucial for cell metabolism.

NAD: NAD stands for Nicotinamide Adenine Dinucleotide. That's a fancy long term for a coenzyme that supports mitochondrial function. Without it, you couldn't produce energy.

Autophagy: Autophagy is the natural, conserved degradation of the cell that removes unnecessary or dysfunctional components. It allows the orderly degradation and recycling of cellular components to help regenerate newer, healthier cells. "Auto" means self and "phagy" means eat, so appropriately, it's self-degradation.

How do all of these things come together to support you? Sirtuins are a class of genes that are instrumental in the body's protection against aging.

- They require NAD+ to do their job (think of NAD+ as sirtuin fuel).
- NAD is an electron/proton acceptor. It helps transfer electrons.
- Metabolism involves taking the energy of chemical bonds in food, breaking them down, and freeing energy up, which is then used to create electrical energy via the electron transport chain.
- NAD+ helps with this transfer of energy.
- As we age, our NAD levels diminish because we make less, and we use more if it.
- The older you get, the more you need the repair benefit of sirtuins.

Sirtuins, which are NAD dependent, help activate the mitochondria in your cell to support NAD. Mitochondria are ancient bacteria that are the energy powerhouses of the cell. They support the cycle of energy.

NAD corrects mitochondrial imbalances, helps transfer energy, and because we make less as we age, we don't repair cells as well.

("Metabolic and Neuropsychiatric Effects of Calorie Restriction and Sirtuins", *Annual Physiology*, 2013.)

Sirtuins mediate a number of metabolic and behavioral responses to calorie restriction.

Downstream effects of calorie restriction include decreases in cancer incidence, the suppression of reproduction, alterations of metabolic functions with increased fat oxidation, alterations of mood (higher degrees of anxiety and susceptibility to depression), increased aggression, and increased DNA repair. Calorie restriction also robustly increases the longevity and health of laboratory animals.

As you can see, it's a mixed bag. We want a decrease in cancer risk, increased longevity, and DNA repair. We obviously don't want suppressed reproductive function (even if we aren't looking to have a child, we want our hormones functioning in a balanced way), and of course, we don't want aggressive "hangry" moods. We've all been there if we've gone too long without eating.

However, there is a way to activate your sirtuins without calorie restriction.

There are six main sirtuins we have discovered and know about. Many more continue to be discovered! We'll refer to them as Sirts below:

- Sirts 1 and 6 suppress inflammation. When you calm down inflammation, you start metabolizing fat and/or building muscle much more effectively.
- Sirt 1 is necessary for optimal brain health.
    - This protects against neurodegenerative diseases and supports a great mood!
- Sirt 3 enhances mitochondrial function and provides better ketone production
    - Burning ketones as a fuel source helps you burn fat as fuel. When people get to a state of ketosis, they feel great, clear energy.
    - We want to enhance this Sirtuin support of our mitochondria!
- Sirt 6 stops fat storage and helps with DNA repair.
    - This occurs with time restricted eating.
    - Sirtuins help to repair or get rid of cells in poor health, replacing them with new stem cells (a.k.a. autophagy!).

What the Heck Does This Have to do With Vegetables?

It's all coming together.

Sirtuins are inherent in many plant-based foods. Imagine, you are getting all the benefits we've described above simply from consuming particular foods, especially vegetables.

Which foods contain sirtuins?

- Quercetin: Plant polyphenols
- Fruits: Wild strawberries, all dark berries, apples, lemons, pomegranates, dates
- Dark cacao powder: 85% or greater with Chocolate
- Spices: turmeric, chili, curry, ginger, cinnamon, capers, cloves, cumin
- Veggies: dark leafy greens, broccoli, artichoke, red onion, celery
- Herbs: parsley, oregano, peppermint, rosemary, thyme, basil
- Drinks (all organic): Coffee, Chamomile (which also has the benefit of L-theanine that helps you sleep at night), Matcha Green Tea, and Red Wine (in very small amounts! If you can't moderate consumption in a sitting and sip on caffeine, wine, or eat just a little piece of chocolate, then utilize these others first.)
- Additionally:
    - Extra Virgin Olive Oil and Olives
    - Glycine from chicken
    - Walnuts
    - Flax

- Buckwheat

You can also increase conversion of white fat to brown fat through consuming mint, curcumin, and green tea. You increase cellular autophagy with a combination of Quercetin, Pau d'Arco, Milk Thistle, Glycine, and Chamomile.

I bet you thought we'd strictly talk about what you've probably already heard: that eating all the colors of the rainbow in vegetables helps support the functionality of your system and overall well-being. Isn't this fascinating to see how much we truly need plants to support health on a deeper, cellular level?

Chewing

Did you know chewing actually supports jaw health in the long run? Consuming too many smoothies or already broken down/mashed foods can actually weaken your jawline over time. Do yourself a favor and get to chewing vegetables!

Cooking

Studies have shown that cooking denatures proteins and makes them more bioavailable.

Researchers have shown that digestibility goes from 51% to 90% when cooked vs. raw.

The energetic benefit of cooking increases bioavailability by approximately 78%.

Challenge Time

1. Eat at least one pound of organic veggies daily, maybe even two pounds. (Make sure they are cooked! That will aid digestion and make it easier to hit the goal. If you have an autoimmune disorder, definitely don't eat cruciferous veggies raw.)

   Ex: Fill up a frying pan with veggies and one-half to one cup of water, and steam them down. Add butter or olive oil, sea salt, seasonings and herbs, sprouts (raw), and enjoy!

2. One day per week, set your intention on food prep!

   Put a grocery list together, put prepped food in nice glass containers, and lay your supplements out. Mason jars can be used to easily prep your veggies and salads. You'll feel so good knowing it's all done!

One to two pounds sounds like a lot, right? Here are several examples, and trust us. When you cook these down, you will hit this goal in no time!

Cruciferous vegetables are great! Examples include broccoli, cauliflower, bok choy, kale, collard greens, and more. Be sure to cook them for easier digestion, especially if you have an autoimmune condition. We are not asking for one to two pounds raw, or you'd be chewing all day long on salads!

Benefits of cruciferous vegetables:

- Reduced risk of cardiovascular disease mortality!
- 51% reduction of bladder cancer!

- Reduction of prostate cancer!
- Reduction of estrogen dominance (decreases risk of breast cancer with just one or two servings a day by 20 to 40%!).
    - Remember, estrogen is fat storing so we want to boost muscle mass and keep fat in check.
    - DIM in these veggies helps this process of estrogen clearance.

Sulforaphane is also inherent in cruciferous vegetables. Sulforaphane is a major anti-inflammatory agent, and helps prevent inflammatory diseases and athrosclorotic diseases. You can get this through sprouts like broccoli sprouts. Don't cook the sprouts. You want to eat them raw.

Additionally, sulforaphane helps with neuropathy. Studies have shown that rats with diabetic neuropathy fed sulforaphane helps change the whole pattern of the disease. If you have nerve damage you need sulforaphane.

Counting

If you don't like counting things, just start putting two handfuls of veggie on your plate (about half the plate) at meals, and include the spices and herbs above. Treat the "treats" like chocolate, caffeinated coffee/tea, and wine as a small bonus.

Do one day of meal prep (or two days during the week if that works better). Cook once, eat two or three times, and spread out your leftovers. Making the decision in advance of what you will eat will make this process so much easier. When the planning and prepping is done, it's time to eat and enjoy!

Here's a helpful chart so you can see how doable this is:

Asparagus	1 pound = 3 cups chopped
Beans (string)	1 pound = 4 cups chopped
Beets	1 pound (5 medium) = 2-½ cups chopped
Broccoli	½ pound = 3 cups chopped
Cabbage	1 pound = 4-½ cups shredded
Carrots	1 pound = 3-½ cups sliced or grated
Celery	1 pound = 4 cups chopped
Cucumbers	1 pound (2 medium) = 4 cups sliced
Eggplant	1 pound = 4 cups chopped (6 cups raw, cubed = 3 cups cooked)
Garlic	1 clove = 1 teaspoon chopped
Leeks	1 pound = 4 cups chopped (2 cups cooked)
Mushrooms	1 pound = 5 to 6 cups sliced = 2 cups cooked
Onions	1 pound = 4 cups sliced = 2 cups cooked
Parsnips	1 pound unpeeled = 1-½ cups cooked and pureed

Peas	1 pound whole = 1 to 1-½ cups shelled
Potatoes	1 pound (3 medium) sliced = 2 cups mashed
Pumpkin	1 pound = 4 cups chopped = 2 cups cooked and drained
Spinach	1 pound = ¾ to 1 cup cooked
Squash (summer)	1 pound = 4 cups grated = 2 cups salted and drained
Squash (winter)	2 pounds = 2-½ cups cooked and pureed
Sweet potatoes	1 pound = 4 cups grated = 1 cup cooked and pureed
Swiss chard	1 pound = 5 to 6 cups packed leaves = 1 to 1-½ cups cooked
Tomatoes	1 pound (3 or 4 medium) = 1-½ cups seeded pulp
Turnips	1 pound = 4 cups chopped = 2 cups cooked and mashed

If you haven't been much of a veggie eater before picking up this book, I promise you, your tastes and what you crave can change! When I noticed a shift from eating junk foods to craving whole foods and vegetables, it was such a great feeling! I love how vegetables make me feel and support my energy and vitality.

One of my favorite meals is sautéed chopped mixed cruciferous vegetables and cauliflower rice, then good quality bacon crumbled on top, and some Kite Hill ricotta cheese added in. If you tolerate dairy, organic cheese is great, too. I love how crunchy, salty, and savory it is.

Hopefully that gets you away from thinking you have to eat boring boiled cabbage on a plate. Not true! There are so many ways to prepare veggies with herbs, seasoning, and clean sauces that make eating veggies fun.

The Carnivore Diet for Trouble Digesting Veggies

For those of you who can't seem to digest vegetables no matter how much you cook them or what variety you try. The next chapter will give you something to try. Just eat one to two pounds of meat daily for 30 days. This gut reset process will need professional oversight, so reach out to me at regan@gowellness.com, and I'm happy to help.

Also check out some of the work of Paul Saladino, MD, and learn more about the science of this diet. His work shows that several plants release small amounts of toxins that an lead to digestive issues, leaky gut, SIBO, and eczema. I personally have done the 30-day meat-only reset and felt great. I have also assisted several patients through this process. Yes, it is controversial, but can be lifesaving.

Up next, we're going to teach you how to gain even more benefits from eating the right foods in the right amounts without ever feeling deprived!

Peptide

MOTS-c, the Mitochondrial Miracle Grow

About a decade ago, researchers discovered the MOTS-c gene expression in Japanese people who lived beyond 100 years of age.
www.ncbi.nlm.nih.gov/pmc/articles/PMC4693465

Not only does MOTS-c promote longevity, but in human and animal studies, it also has been shown to help with muscle growth and protect against insulin resistance, metabolism, heart, liver, and inflammation. MOTS-c mediates mitochondrial regulation of insulin sensitivity and metabolic homeostasis. It protects against age and diet-dependent insulin resistance and obesity.

MOTS-c is the closest thing that researchers have found that mimics exercise and as this gene is expressed more in people who exercise. The use of this as a supplement to your program is a great idea.

Chapter Thirteen
Protein

PROTEIN

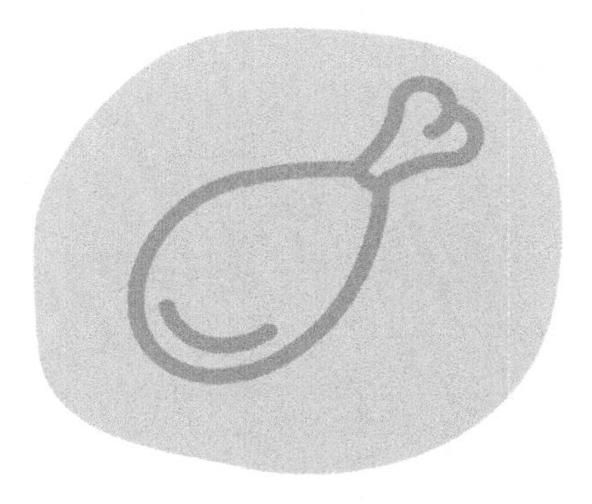

Reverse Dieting

Mindset Twelve
Muscles keep me fit and burning fat, animal proteins allow me to build and keep muscle on.

Our aim throughout this book, and what we want you to take away more than anything with *Never Stop Healing*, is to get 1% better each day, every day.

Let's check in! You've already accomplished implementing 12 different habits! What changes are you noticing? What do you think is having the greatest impact?

Take some time to write those down and don't forget to celebrate your wins! It's so easy to overlook them and how far you've come. The brain easily focuses on the negative, but being grateful towards yourself for all your hard work and effort and showing up for yourself every day can reset your mindset like no other. Practicing gratitude towards yourself is welcomed and encouraged because you are here, doing the work. Bravo!

I'm excited for you, because this one challenge had a huge impact on me many years ago when I was in my 20s. I was a calorie counter back in the day, and while it would work for a time to be rigorously tracking calories, it never felt sustainable. In focusing on the limited number of calories I allotted myself, my brain felt just that: limited, restricted, and deprived. I resented the practice. I would fight the urge to eat more with all the willpower I could muster until I'd eventually (inevitably) give up and binge eat. As you already know (and may have experienced yourself), it just didn't work.

I did an intense six-week boot camp within my first year living in NYC. I wanted to test my limits and see how fit I could get if I truly dedicated myself to it. It was easy to get and stay in phenomenal shape while moving non-stop in college classes, but I was still adjusting to living in the Big Apple.

While calories were a part of it, for the first time, I was taught the power of filling up those calories with super nutrient dense macronutrients, in high amounts. It wasn't just "hit this calorie goal". I was tasked with eating my bodyweight in grams of protein, along with a set number of fats and carbohydrates per day.

I had always been petite, but eating my body weight in grams of protein felt like a LOT! How would I fit it all in?

To my amazement, after just the first two weeks, I started to notice the difference around my waist and was seeing definition in my stomach by the end of the six weeks. While I was working out six days a week, cardio on off days and three days of intense strength training, I thought I'd be ravenous and dissatisfied on another restricted calorie diet (1,200 to 1,500 range). Because I was eating plenty of protein, veggies, and fat throughout the day, though, I could "eat less" and feel full.

I'd have eggs in the morning with veggies mixed in and be satisfied for hours. This replaced my oatmeal at the time. I'd have a big grilled chicken salad most nights. While I did pile up on dairy to help me reach that goal (I wasn't a health coach yet, and boy, did I love cheese, cottage cheese, and greek yogurt), I was a lean, mean, burning machine.

It was very informative. I took away from that experience that it's not just how much you eat that matters. It's the quality of what you eat and macronutrient ratios.

While I don't currently count it gram for gram, I do eat as much grass-fed beef, quality steak, wild-caught salmon, and roasted free-range chicken I want. I feel better energy with great protein on my plate. My friends know me as a "cavewoman". When you put me in front of an organic roasted chicken, I'll clean the meat off the bones!

Now you may be thinking, "I thought I'm supposed to be vegan! I thought meat causes cancer!" Neither of these is true when it comes to high quality meat, and we will teach you what that means.

However, if you choose to not eat animal protein for religious reasons, for your love of animals, or you don't feel well when you eat them, we are not here to judge. There are many plant foods that can serve as great protein sources.

Just please keep in mind that if you are eating a vegan/vegetarian diet and you are lethargic, bloated, overweight, and dealing with a host of hormonal, digestive, skin, and/or other conditions, it's time to revamp and get some help with your diet. We are happy to do that with you one-to-one and meet you where you are.

You'll also learn that we are not advocates for factory farmed meat, poultry, eggs, fish, or processed animal products whatsoever. More on that later.

If you are skeptical that protein can help you, keep reading. We're here to give you the facts on why this macro is so important to achieving optimal health.

Why Yo-Yo Dieting Doesn't Work

["Weight in U.S. Adults who Experienced Substantial Weight Loss". *American Journal of Preventive Medicine,* Data analyzed from 1999–2002 by the National Health and Nutrition Examination Survey (NHANES).]

This study examined U.S. adults ages 20 to 84, who were overweight or obese at their maximum weight (body mass index ≥ 25) and had experienced substantial weight loss (weighed 10% less than their maximum weight one year before they were surveyed) (*n* = 1,310).

Results:

- Compared to their weight one year ago, 7.6% had continued to lose weight (>5%).
- 58.9% had maintained their weight (within 5%).
- 33.5% had regained weight (>5%).

Weight regain was higher in those who were sedentary (OR = 1.8; 95% CI = 1.0–3.0) or not meeting public health recommendations for physical activity (OR = 2.0; 95% CI = 1.2–3.5).

Conclusions: Creating new skills necessary for long-term maintenance of weight loss in the context of an obesogenic environment remains a challenge.

How is your environment, your community and support? Who are you helping throughout this process?

I want to take a moment to really hone in on why this is so important.

Just as children emulate their parents, we end up consciously (or unconsciously) picking up on and participating in the habits of those we spend the most time with. Now's the time to create great habits for yourself and be the example you wish to see for kids, your loved ones, friends, etc. Choose your community and spend time with people who celebrate your desire to be the best you want to be!

Simultaneously, when you are in the midst of changing old habits into new, that process is not easy! There will be mental resistance, and if you are not surrounded by a group who supports what you are doing, it's so easy to feel left out and want to throw in the towel.

Not to mention that some give up on their health goals out of a deeper fear over abandonment, no longer feeling loved, or other emotional belief system surrounding their old identity. The unconscious fear that says by changing, any of that could be true, would cause any sane person to sabotage their best efforts consciously or unconsciously. Beliefs have a powerful influence.

Continuously going to events with people who don't understand your desire to be healthy, don't support it, and/or try to push foods on you can be exhausting. (Trust us, we know.) While we can't always escape family gatherings, we can learn to have solid habits and become less triggered by the choices of other people around us. We can also learn to question our own beliefs and come back to our why statement to lock in the habit, even in the midst of temptations.

Just because someone else is eating cake doesn't mean you have to. It doesn't mean you need to. It doesn't mean you'll offend them if you don't, and if you do, that's not on you, AND it doesn't mean you'll be left out of the fun or have to feel deprived.

Question ALL the belief systems that come up, especially around communal eating and celebrations. Question what it really means to enjoy yourself at an event and connect with others and what you can do to support that ultimate goal.

If you don't feel comfortable sharing the changes you are making or know that others aren't ready to hear it, that's good to take note of. Set healthy boundaries. Eventually, we'd love for you to share everything you are learning and growing from, but some people aren't ready for change.

As you learned in the beginning of this book, we discussed how setting up your environment is so crucial for habits, and the study above proves it!

If you are someone who craves accountability and understands the power of community and connection with habit change, please come join our Online Health Accelerator Challenge group! You can go to www.acueastwest.com/hac to learn how it works, and join the live weekly coaching sessions at www.acueastwest.com/hac-launch.

We also have a private texting channel on Signal that you are welcome to become a part of. We share resources, wins, challenges, and support one another's growth! The group is overseen, moderated, and supported by a Health Coach and Regan.

Seeking help on your journey and reminding yourself you don't have to go about this alone or "figure it all out" or "know all the answers" by yourself is such a relief. We are meant to help one another and receive help when needed. The journey is 10 times more enjoyable when we do. Come join us!

Calories In, Calories Out

How many of you have heard the phrase, "Calories in, Calories out?" This refers to the need to reduce calories taken in and increase expenditure via exercise if you want to lose weight. The opposite is therefore recommended if you want to gain weight, and to maintain, ensure that you burn what you take in every day. One pound burned or gained can equal 3,500 calories, depending on your expenditure.

While quantity does matter, this simple equation doesn't work across the board for weight loss. It oversimplifies and doesn't take into consideration the vast number of functions that, if thrown off track, won't permit your body to lose or gain even if you use this formula perfectly.

Take a look at this awesome infographic to better understand the many ways that different functions of the body affect energy intake and expenditure.

FACTORS THAT INFLUENCE ENERGY

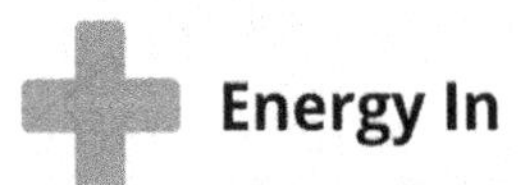

Energy In

Appetite

Hormones influence appetite + satiety

Foods Consumed

Availability, palatability, energy density, sleep quality, education, socioeconomic status, culture

Calories Absorbed

Macro intake, food prep, age, personal microbiome, health status, energy status

Psychological Factors

Stress levels, mindset, perceived control, self-esteem, sleep quality

Energy Out

Energy Burned at Rest

Body size, hormone status, dieting history, genetics, health status, sleep quality, age

Energy Burned in Exercise

Exercise ability, intensity, duration, frequency, type, environment, hormonal status, sleep quality

Energy Burned by Non-Exercise Activity

Health status, energy status, stress levels, hormone status, occupation, leisure activities, genetic factors

Energy Burned Metabolizing Food

Macronutrient makeup, disease, microbiome health, how food is processed

While this isn't a comprehensive list, it helps you gain an understanding of how many factors can influence your ability to lose weight or why you gain weight. This doesn't even include medications or the influence of different diseases or functional breakdown.

Are you ready to finally let go of this outdated advice and embrace a new way of eating?

Yo-Yo Dieting vs. Reverse Dieting

As you saw in the study at the beginning of this chapter, restricting calories for a period of time and losing weight, only to go back to what you ate before causes you to "Yo-Yo", gaining all the weight back (and then some!).

Yo-yo dieting does the opposite of what we actually want in terms of results.

- Your basal metabolic rate declines in proportion to calorie deficit (the amount of energy you need when at rest).
- Your ability to burn fat weakens.
- You become anxious, irritable, exhausted, and hungry at all hours of the day.
- You expend LESS energy through exercise!
- You won't be able to get to the next level of your fitness potential and strength.
- Your body goes into conservation mode. Especially for women, this can throw off your cycle and your body's ability to conceive. Your body is in a stressed state and doesn't prioritize fertility.

This is not the same as Time Restricted Eating. Remember the rat study? The rats ate the same number of calories in the TRE group and the control group. They only restricted the time frame in which the rats ate those calories five days a week.

While fasting does give your body a break from food, and we can last a lot longer without food than we can without clean water and air, it's important to remember that surviving and thriving are not the same thing. You can eat a reasonable number of high-density macronutrients, feel satisfied and not starved, and still lose weight.

You can stop the vicious cycle of yo-yo dieting and calorie counting, and we're going to teach you how with something called "Reverse Dieting".

Reverse Dieting is increasing your calories (in this case, through protein) in order to increase metabolism, increase muscle mass, and simultaneously decrease body fat.

Reverse dieting helps you:

- Maintain weight loss.
- Maintain metabolic rate over time.
- Helps you burn fat.

The goal of a reverse diet or "recovery diet" is to increase your metabolic efficiency and to mitigate and reverse the adaptations that were done due to the caloric restriction.

homebase.org/news/nutrition-reverse-dieting-101/

Let's Talk Macros!

Macronutrients are inherent in every food and fall into one of three categories: Carbohydrates, Proteins, and Fats. Check out any nutrition label, and while some foods may be only two of the three or the majority, one of the three, you will find some combination of macronutrients in every single food.

Eating what's called "Nutrient Dense" food offers good quality macros in healthy amounts per serving, along with great micronutrients: chemical elements or substances required in trace amounts for the normal growth and development of living organisms. Think Vitamins and Minerals. We need both components to thrive.

How do you know how much you currently eat?

Rather than counting calories, I like this visual depiction of assessing general serving sizes (portions) of macronutrients using your hand on the go! No scales or extensive tracking necessary.

See each of these depictions as a good visual gauge for one serving size of each of those macronutrients. (Veggies are mostly carbs, but don't worry about overeating your veggies right now. As shown in the last challenge, we want you to eat one to two pounds!)

Use this at restaurants, when making your plate at home, at a party, etc. When it comes to protein, we'll share at the end the amount you are aiming for.

PORTIONS BY HAND

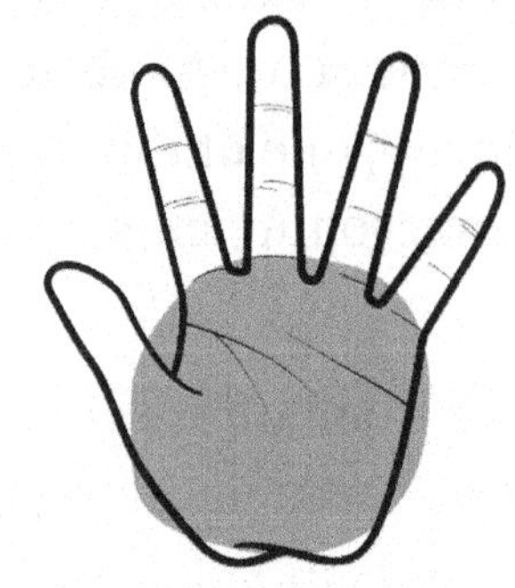

1 Portion Protein = the size of your palm

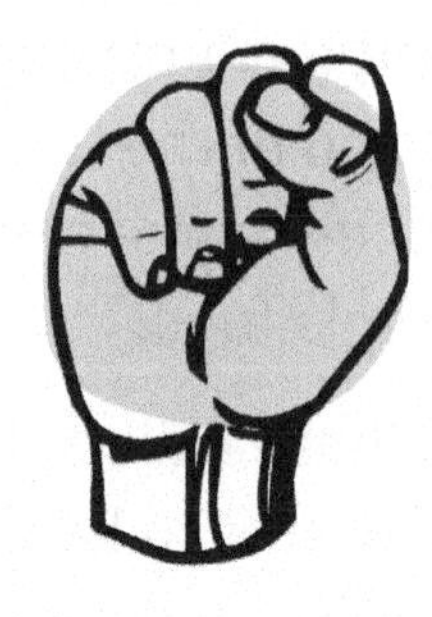

1 Portion Veggies = your closed fist

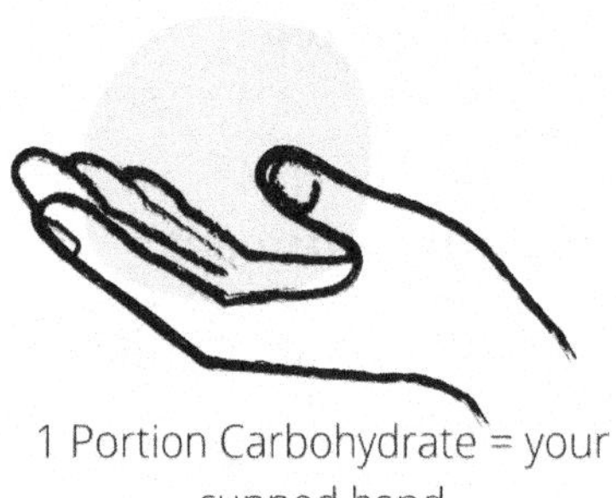

1 Portion Carbohydrate = your cupped hand

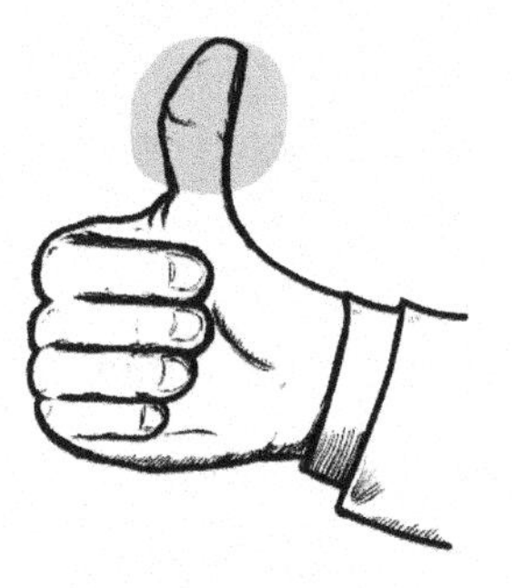

1 Portion Fat = your thumb

If you do like to track, we'll be aiming for grams, so let's go through a quick lesson on how to measure grams of protein and serving sizes. (If you prefer not to track this way, that's okay! Do what works best for you.)

Seven grams of protein is about one serving size. Three or four servings in a sitting comes out to about 21 to 30 grams. While that might seem like a lot, given the typical portions of food are already much larger than the size of your palm, dense protein sources can quickly add up to well above 30 grams in a sitting! (Just don't stuff yourself.

Eat slowly and consciously so you give your body time to break it down and signal you are full.)

Clean carbohydrates are foods like gluten free cooled rice, cooled potatoes, sweet potatoes, other gluten free grains like quinoa and whole foods that are mostly carbohydrates. Fifteen grams of carbs equal one serving. While veggies are mostly carbohydrates, we want you to aim for one to one and a half pounds of non-starchy veggies.

For other whole foods that are mostly carbs per above, aim for one or two servings max in a sitting. If you are active/have a great metabolism you may feel better with more. If you have a metabolic issue, diabetes, other disease, or microbiome imbalances that thrive on carbohydrate rich foods, you need to be a bit more restrictive. Talk to a functional medicine provider to gain more clarity as to the best amount for you. If you want a gram range, try 50 g (which is on the much lower end of only three servings) to 120 g (which is eight servings and on the higher end).

We'll talk more towards the end of this chapter about how much we are aiming for per day (both in general servings and grams so you can choose which method you use to track).

Not All Proteins Are Created Equal

What you are probably used to seeing on shelves and hearing about in the news and in documentaries is about mass production of meat killing our planet. Not to mention the gruesome treatment of animals you may have seen in those documentaries that walk you through the conditions of factory farms.

When I say, "Factory Farmed meat," I'm not talking about animals grazing out in wide-open green fields, well-fed and well-treated, with lots of fresh air and sunshine. Factory farming creates disease and bacteria infested breeding grounds where animals are kept in such close proximity that every square inch of the barn is covered.

Without any space, living in their own filth, animals can easily develop diseases and infections. One would think that would mean the entire animal is deemed useless for human consumption, but they treat the animals or in some instances simply "cut around" diseased portions to cut corners.

If any animals have a bacterial infection, they are fed antibiotics (just like humans) which we later ingest when we eat the animal. Are you grossed out yet? There's more.

Factory farmed animals are also fed growth hormones to make them bigger, increasing their size for more money earned per animal. They are fed grains to make them fatter (to enhance flavor), and are severely abused and mistreated. Factory farmed meat, poultry, and fish is definitely not the kind of high-quality meat and protein we are talking about here.

The type of meat, poultry, eggs, and fish we recommend eating have certain designations. Upon doing a little refresher research on how to interpret labels, I'm finding many claims are not as clear-cut as they would seem, but I've done my best to outline it for you so you know what each label means.

At the end of the day, going to your local farmers' market and getting to know the practices of your chosen farm is truly what's best to know for certain. There are helpful questions to ask your farmer included in these blog posts as well.

The below notes came from articles by The Real Food Dieticians I found very informative:

- therealfooddietitians.com/understanding-poultry-labels/
- therealfooddietitians.com/how-to-choose-quality-red-meat/
- therealfooddietitians.com/how-to-choose-safer-seafood/

Meat:

- **Certified Organic:** "Seeing the 'USDA Organic' label on your meat is great, but it only tells part of the story. Under organic standards, meat can be labeled organic if the animal received at least 30% of its diet from grass or dried forage. The remaining part of the diet, if comprised of grains, would have had to have been organic grains. Also, to be considered organic, the animal must not have received growth hormones or antibiotics. (Note: Antibiotics are used in organic farming but only when absolutely necessary to save the life of a sick animal that, after treatment, would no longer qualify as organic.)
- **Grass-Fed and Grass Finished:** There are currently no government standards for grass-fed

meat, so look for labels from third-party organizations that say "PCO Certified", "100% Grass-Fed", or "American Grass-Fed". If you'd like to dive deeper into why it's important to eat grass-fed and not grain-fed meat, please check out the helpful articles above.

- **No Growth Hormones or Antibiotics Used on the Animals:** This is inherent in organic, but if non-organic, then look for that distinction.
- **Non-GMO Feed:** GMO stands for Genetically Modified. The use of GMOs is prohibited when organic.
- **No artificial flavors/additives.**
- **Nitrate Free (for bacon, turkey bacon, etc.):** Usually found in processed meats to affect color and taste.
- ****Free-range** only applies to chicken by regulations.

Poultry/Eggs:

- **Organic Certified:** This term is regulated by the USDA and ensures that all feed (that the animals are fed) must be certified organic and free of animal by-products, synthetic fertilizers, pesticides, or other additives such as hormones or antibiotics. USDA organic standards also require that poultry must meet "free-range" criteria as well.

- **Free-Range/Free-Roaming/Cage-Free:** "It's important to note that the United States Department of Agriculture (USDA) only allows the term 'free-range' to be used for chicken and not for eggs or other animals (such as cattle, pigs, or sheep). For chickens to be considered 'free-range,' they must have access to the outdoors each day for an undetermined amount of time. While this would imply that the birds are freely roaming in nature, soaking up the sun, and eating their natural diet of grasses and bugs, there are currently no regulatory agencies overseeing this to be sure that's actually what's happening. That means they could spend most of their lives outdoors, retreating to their coop only when weather conditions warrant doing so, or they could spend their entire lives in cramped, overcrowded indoor conditions with a small door that opens to the outside for only a few minutes each day. The regulation only states that they 'must have daily access to the outdoor', so the only way to know how your chicken spent its days is to ask and do your research."
- **Certified Humane:** "This term is not regulated by the USDA, but is instead overseen by a nonprofit organization called Humane Farm Animal Care who ensure that the birds receive certain basic standards of care and are allowed (and encouraged) to participate in normal poultry behaviors such as roaming, scratching, pecking, perching, and foraging for food in their bedding."

- **Pasture-Raised:** This is also an unregulated term, but the Humane Farm Animal Care group has established a standard which states that, to be "pasture-raised," birds must be raised outdoors year-round with access to shelter to protect them from weather and predators.
- **Non-GMO Feed**
- **Vegetarian Feed** means they haven't been fed animal byproducts, but it doesn't mean they were given free-range access to eating outdoors.
- **Hormones** aren't allowed to be used on chicken.
- **Antibiotic Free:** "This term can only be legally used when the producer is able to produce significant documentation to the FSIS that the chicken or turkey was in fact produced without the administration of antibiotics (whether used to treat illness or used prophylactically in feed or water to prevent disease)."

Fish:

- Larger fish tend to contain higher **mercury** levels, so to avoid, it's best not to eat shark, tilefish, king mackerel, bluefin ahi tuna, swordfish, or Atlantic flatfish such as halibut, flounder, and sole.
- Make sure it's **Wild-Caught** and never "Farm Raised"
- **A note about preservatives:** Shrimp often has preservatives added to it during processing. Look

for words like Sodium Tripolyphosphate (STPP) or Trisodium Phosphate (TSP), sodium bisulfate, and "Everfresh". Though considered "safe" by the FDA, they can have adverse health effects including sensitivity, excess sodium content, and possibly even exposure to xenoestrogens in the case of Everfresh. It's best to choose those without additives whenever possible.

- Helpful resources provided by **The Real Food Dieticians** to help you choose sustainable, clean fish:
    - Environmental Defense Fund Seafood Selector
        - Includes info for mercury, environmental concerns and recommended servings per month for each species. This is their favorite resource.
    - Monterey Bay Aquarium's Seafood Watch Guide
        - Available as a handy printable wallet card or searchable online database.
    - Marine Stewardship Council
        - Learn more about sustainable fishing and what this label and certification means on the seafood you buy.
    - Aquaculture Stewardship Council

- Use their product locator (set country filter to "United States" or other desired country) to get a list of certified seafood brands and products.

For all of the above, EWG (Environmental Working Group) is also a helpful resource to stay informed of changes: www.ewg.org

Some great organizations you can order from for delivery of clean meat, poultry, and fish include Butcher Box and Vital Choice.

Additional Sources of Protein to your Diet

Some of Regan's favorite protein sources include bison meat and liver, while mine include 100% grass-fed beef and organic roasted chicken with the skin. I also love wild-caught salmon.

While animal products are packed with protein, you can also get protein added to your goal through vegetables and carbohydrates (varies per food). Even foods that contain mostly healthy fats can have some protein content as well. It will all add up and contribute to your goal! This is actually why it can be helpful to have an app to track grams for you when you input what you eat so that you truly see how much total protein each meal contains.

Certain Veggies have good protein content per serving:

- Brussels Sprouts
- Asparagus

- Spinach (It shrinks when you cook a cup, so you can eat a lot more cooked in one sitting!)
- Broccoli
- Sprouts
- Artichokes
- Collards
- Winter Squash
- Natto (You don't want to consume too much of other types of soy like edamame as it can throw your hormones off. Definitely no processed soy!)

Other helpful sources beyond meat, fish, poultry, and eggs include:

- Colostrum (great for gut health)
- Collagen Powder (great for skin and connective tissue)
- Whey Protein (if you want to bulk up)
- Pea Protein (if this causes you gut issues, your body may be responding poorly to lectins so you can pull that out and try a different option above)
- Organic High-Quality Dairy (goat's milk can be better tolerated)
- Bone Broth

High Protein for Fat Burning

("Higher Dietary Protein Intake Is Associated with Lower Body Fat in the Newfoundland Population", *Journal Of Endocrinology*, 2010.)

This study involved a total of 1,834 participants.

Results:

- Significant inverse relationships were observed between dietary protein intake (g/kg body weight/day) and weight, waist circumference, waist-to-hip ratio, BMI, %BF, and %TF ($P < 0.001$).
- Significant positive relationships were observed with %LM and %TLM ($P < 0.001$). Additionally, significant differences in weight (12.7 kg in men, 11.4 kg in women), BMI (4.1 BMI units in men, 4.2 units in women), and %BF (7.6% in men, 6.0% in women) were observed between low and high dietary protein consuming groups ($P < 0.001$).
- Dietary protein explained 11% of the total variation in %BF in the NL population.

Conclusion: This study provides strong evidence that higher protein intake, even in the absence of energy restriction, is associated with a more favorable body composition in the general population.

A higher protein diet seems to maximize muscle protein synthesis and minimize protein breakdown, which should lead to more muscle gain. This is probably one of the reasons higher protein diets are better for improving body composition than moderate or low protein diets.

Depending on your activity levels, about one to two grams of protein per pound is ideal.

Here's an example: For fat loss for a 160-lb, 42-year-old male who is very active, that equates to 200 to 240 grams/day (closer to 240 if he's trying to gain muscle mass).

For a 60-year-old female who is 5'6",160 lbs. and moderately active who wants to burn fat, she will need about 160 grams of protein.

When you have more muscle, you burn fat more effectively and have a higher metabolism!

With reverse dieting, we are building up muscle mass and metabolic conditioning to help our bodies adjust. We are looking at protein selectively based on the qualities above.

How Do I know How Many G*rams* of Protein I'm Getting?

As mentioned, seven grams of protein equal one full serving of protein, and you can find the amount on nutrition labels of food. With whole foods that don't have labels, you can Google search the general nutrition information for specific foods.

Keep in mind food labels can be off by as much as 20 to 25%. That's not to discourage you, and we aren't looking for perfection. Just do your best to eye it with your hands to know about how many servings you've had in a day. Your goal to start will be 150 g = 21.5 servings at seven grams per serving. Broken down into three to four meals that's about 30 to 40 grams per meal.

If you do like things to be calculated for you to the gram, you can download a tracking app like *Lose It* or *My Fitness Pal*. Do your best to scan barcodes/utilize nutrition labels for your entries that reflect what is on the package. Some are entered by users and aren't accurate but you'll quickly pick up on what works.

Certain apps like *Lose It* also give you a pie chart to read your macros. You can enter your goal for each macro group and see how each meal and each day adds up. You can also save meals and carry them over to other days so you aren't having to enter information individually every day. I used this method when doing the six-week boot camp to track my grams of protein per day, and it was extremely helpful and easy.

We're not using calories to count here, as the amount of energy a food contains in calories is not reflective of the exact amount we absorb, store, and use. We're focusing on macros.

Your Challenge: We are recommending you do 150 grams of protein per day as your initial goal. See how it feels, and be SURE you have read and done the "Love Your Liver" challenge, "Optimize Your Gut" Challenge, and "Veggies" challenge prior to increasing your protein.

Make sure you have adequate digestive enzymes, probiotics, and prebiotics to stay "regular". Too much animal protein and not enough vegetables and fiber can lead to constipation. You should be having a healthy bowel movement at least once per day.

Try to eat liver, heart, or other organ meats at least once per week to balance out your methionine production. Feel free to take capsules if you aren't feeling adventurous enough yet. Eating animal fats is great for you, and ideally, they will be included in the protein sources you are munching on.

If you are eating quality meat and feeling weighed down, sluggish, or dealing with digestive upset, it might not be the meat. It could be a sign your digestive system is not primed to break down proteins or is sluggish for other reasons. That's where a detox is great and supporting your gut with all of Regan's healing tools in *Your Health Transformation*.

By the way, as you've seen throughout this chapter, we aren't recommending you go on the Carnivore diet, Atkins, or any other generic fad meat-based diet. Simply follow the guidelines we've laid out to understand how excellent protein intake positively changes your physique! Enjoy "Reverse Dieting"!

Peptides

Better Protein Absorption with KPV

KPV is a tri-peptide that naturally exists in your small intestine. Its key role is calming inflammation. Studies show that, in the presence of KPV, mice with colitis experience a remission of symptoms. www.ncbi.nlm.nih.gov/pmc/articles/PMC5498804

KPV can help eradicate any infections that may have come from improper digestion of your fats, proteins, or vegetables. It can also aid in eliminating Lyme, Epstein Barr virus, or any chronic viral infections through the melano-corticoid system.

Chapter Fourteen
Fat

FAT

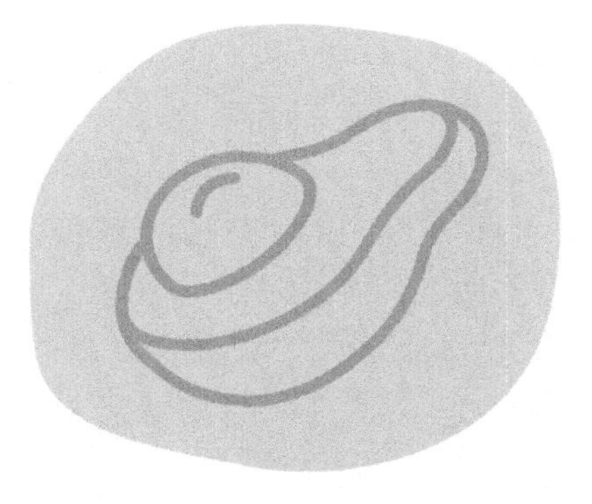

Eat Fat, Get Slim

Mindset Thirteen
While I've been taught the opposite for a long time, it's safe and great to eat different forms of healthy fat!

You made it! This is your final habit in the 100-Day Body Reset. Peptides are a bonus that we hope you'll explore further with us.

How do you feel? What are your wins from the whole experience? We'd love to hear about them! Please contact us and let us know your success with the HAC book. As mentioned, join the community live, online where we are providing ongoing education and support! www.acueastwest.com/hac

As a recap, here are five major ingredient groups to avoid in your diet:

- Refined and added sugars
- Bleached/refined flour
- Industrial plant oils (i.e., canola, sunflower, safflower, corn, soy)
- Any artificial ingredients
- Gluten, Dairy, Soy, Corn, Peanuts

These foods create inflammation. We've been building up your body week by week to support using an alternative energy source to glucose/sugar.

Speaking of sugar, how are you doing with getting off the sugar train? Are you still on track? If you've gotten a bit off track since the introduction of our Sugar challenge, just take note. Are there emotional or physical stressors going on? Can you replace sugar with low glycemic fruit and use stevia or monk fruit as your sweetener starting today?

Even I catch myself at times letting sugar sneak back in and have to pull back. I know it's a slippery slope.

Let's go over the top reasons this is so important.

We all want a healthy immune system, robust stem cells, and anti-aging. However, consuming sugar weakens our stem cells and progresses aging.

Excess sugar also depresses immunity, which is more important than ever at this time in history. Studies have shown that downing 75 to 100 grams of a sugar solution (about 20 teaspoons of sugar, or the amount that is contained in two average 12-ounce sodas) can suppress the body's immune responses. Simple sugars, including glucose, table sugar, fructose, and honey caused a 50% drop in the ability of white blood cells to engulf bacteria! academic.oup.com/ajcn/article-abstract/26/11/1180/4732762

Sugar even puts your immune system into a temporary coma.

The immune suppression was most noticeable two hours post-ingestion, but the effect was still evident *five hours after ingestion.* This research has practical implications, especially for teens and college students who tend to overdose on sodas containing caffeine and sugar while studying for exams or during periods of stress. Stress also suppresses immunity, so these sugar users are setting themselves up to get sick at a time when they need to be well.

blog.bioticsresearch.com/does-sugar-weaken-the-immune-system

Cutting out sugar and low-quality dairy significantly boosted my immune system, so I stopped catching every illness after college. I was so resistant at first, but who wants to be sick all the time? I finally place the health of my "future self" over the short-term gratification of gluten, dairy, sugar, and so many other junk foods I used to consume as a kid.

Remember the "fat makes you fat" craze that isn't true?! During that time when we were made to believe fat is the culprit of weight gain, diet foods hit the shelves. With them came an influx of higher sugar because fat makes foods taste good, so sugar took its place. Whether regular, processed, or artificial sugars, a lot of damage was done.

I definitely got on board with "fat free, sugar-free" products in college, and filled my coffee cup with Splenda every morning, or I always ordered "skinny girl lattes" from Starbucks with skim milk and a couple pumps of fake flavored sweeteners. Years later, after transitioning away from that life entirely, I once accidentally consumed something with Splenda that made me grimace. My taste buds have evolved tremendously.

Fast food consumption is also causing dysbiosis and gut inflammation. This further suppresses the immune system, so we're not isolating sugar as the only immune suppressant ingredient on the market.
www.ncbi.nlm.nih.gov/pmc/articles/PMC4074336/

With the rise of our junk food nation has come a deficiency of many vital micronutrients, including fatty acids. This, too, has boosted inflammation, and with it, conditions like Irritable Bowel Disease. *(Int. Rev. Immunol. 2009; 28: 506–53.)*

By the way, wouldn't it be interesting if, instead of calling a disease by its present-day medical name, we called it by its cause? Type II Diabetes could become "Sugar Overconsumption". Cardiovascular Disease could be "Junk Food Carb Addiction" or "Sedentary Lifestyle Syndrome". The brain would go from feeling victim of a diagnosis to realizing what needs to be done.

Not getting enough healthy fats and fatty acids, especially Omega-3s, disrupts our hormone pathways and amplifies inflammation. The majority of junk foods are higher in Omega-6 from sources like industrial oils, corn, and soy, which throws off our balance of Omegas. Omega-3 is very anti-inflammatory and comes from sources like chia seeds, fatty wild caught fish like salmon, cod liver, flax seeds, and walnuts.

Healthy Fats and Your Brain

Your brain loves them! How great that we get to eat healthy fats that taste delicious and boost our brain power.

Your brain is the most fat and cholesterol-dense part of your body, and it requires saturated fat to build myelin, the insulators that connect many of your brain cells to one another. Low-fat diets will starve your brain.

The brain is made of about 57% fat, 38% protein, and contains very little carbohydrate (5%). Our modern brains grew up in a low glycemic index environment.

Even cholesterol is very important for hormonal health and brain health. We don't want too much of it, but we need enough to support the system to do what it's meant to do. Cholesterol builds up the insulators, so your cells fire and wire better.

Regan credits implementing fat in his diet many years ago as saving his brain, having experienced many concussions growing up.

Have you ever wondered why walnuts look like a brain? So many foods in nature are reflective of the organs they support. It's wild. Similarly, the insides of larger carrots look like eyes, sweet potatoes look like the pancreas, celery is long like bones, and grapefruit look similar to breasts when cut in half. All of those foods protect and support the very body parts they resemble!

Healthy Fats Satisfy

Fats are also satiating. No more hunger! If you have eaten and feel hungry soon after, had adequate protein and vegetables, and you have had enough water, did you check to be sure you added healthy fat to your meal? This happened to me when making smoothies. I noticed if I just had protein powder with a little stevia, fruit, and nut milk, I wasn't satisfied! Adding in a tablespoon of nut butter did the trick.

Long-term caloric restriction can stress your body and contribute to leptin resistance, insulin resistance, low testosterone, and thyroid issues, which is why so many people lose weight in the short-term, then gain it all back when they begin to eat normally again. It can also lead you to feeling tired all the time. Fats give you a more sustainable source of energy to pull from.

Satiate your body and brain with good fats, and your cravings will disappear.

Micronutrients

Quality fats often contain fat-soluble vitamins like A, D, E, and K. Those are very important micronutrients on so many levels! Think immune health, skin, hair, and nail health, bone health, eye health, and more.

Eating fat alongside other nutrient-dense foods will increase the fat-soluble nutrients you absorb from them, too. That's why it's a good idea to eat fat at every meal, and especially with your vegetables. It's also why you should consume a multivitamin that contains A, E, D, and/or Vitamin K with a healthy fat to help it absorb properly.

Your Cells & Hormones

Quality fats form strong cell membranes and support cell integrity.

They also help build sex hormones. That means healthier cycles and fertility, and healthier energy and sex drive for males and females alike!

Fats Stabilize Blood Sugar

Fat slows the absorption of carbohydrates, keeping blood glucose levels under control. When blood sugar is high, so is cortisol, your body's main stress hormone. Circulating cortisol will keep blood sugar high and can contribute to inflammation and hurt your immune system. ("Effect of Dietary Fat on Blood Sugar Levels and Insulin Consumption After Intake of Various Carbohydrate Carriers in Type I Diabetics on the Artificial Pancreas." *Int. Journal of Obesity Related Metabolic Disorders*. 1996, May 20.)

Fats Help You Lose Weight!

In a study where two groups of participants consumed the same amount of calories, the group which had more calories from fatty almonds lost the most weight. When it comes down to it, all nuts will be great sources of monounsaturated, polyunsaturated, and omega-3 fats, just in varying amounts. A total of 84 grams of almonds helped, which is just 23 almonds! Just keep in mind peanuts are not actually a nut but, rather, a legume and should be avoided. [*Int J Obes Relat Metab Disorders*. 2003, Nov 27(11)]

If you have a thyroid condition, Regan warns to not overdo it on daily consumption of almonds as they can be harder to digest and harder on the thyroid. Just eat a variety of nuts or alternate, and you'll be good!

Sources of Healthy Fat

Eat the Yolk!

Eggs are a solid source of healthy fat. If you're someone who is still unsure if you should eat the yolk, here's your answer: Yes!

While the whites are all protein, leaving the yolk to contain the fat and cholesterol, there's no need to worry.

Fat in yolks are mostly monounsaturated, and a study by University of Connecticut researchers found that the overall fat profile in egg yolks ultimately helps to reduce LDL ("bad" cholesterol). Above and beyond improving your cholesterol, eggs are the number-one dietary source of a nutrient called choline.

Choline, which is found also in lean meats, seafood, and collard greens, attacks the gene mechanism that triggers your body to store fat around your liver.

Regan loves to cook eggs with butter in a waffle maker so he can easily make a large batch and take them to work! There are so many easy-to-make egg dishes now, like homemade omelets with lots of veggies, baking fluffy eggs in muffin tins for on-the-go mini quiche, or simply hard boiled and thrown on a salad! Mix it up and have fun!

www.eatthis.com/should-i-eat-egg-yolks

academic.oup.com/jn/article/138/2/272/4664988

www.eatthis.com/foods-to-lower-cholesterol

Olive Oil and Adiponectin

Olive oil is rich in cancer-fighting polyphenols and heart-strengthening monounsaturated fats, including oleic acid.

A recent study from *Obesity* found that an olive-oil-rich diet resulted in higher levels of adiponectin than did a high-carb or high-protein diet.
www.ncbi.nlm.nih.gov/pmc/articles/PMC3045829/

Adiponectin is a hormone responsible for breaking down fats in the body.

Olive oil may also increase blood levels of serotonin, a hormone associated with satiety, calm, and happiness.

Just be sure your olive oil is real and not mixed with other unhealthy oils. More and more, even olive oils are being misrepresented and mislabeled because it's not illegal to mix it up, so you aren't always receiving pure, 100% organic extra virgin olive oil. You can check out this site to feel better about your choice of olive oil brand: www.aboutoliveoil.org.

It's ideal to use olive oil raw on a salad or over already cooked veggies as it can't withstand high heat and has a lower smoke point. Think Mediterranean style with your olive oil use.

Cuckoo for Coconuts

Coconut is high in saturated fat. More than half of that comes from lauric acid, a unique medium-chain triglyceride that battles bacteria, improves cholesterol scores, and as a *Journal of Nutrition* study found, increases 24-hour energy expenditure in humans by as much as 5%. academic.oup.com/jn/article/132/3/329/4687297

Lauric acid can be really supportive for yeast infections/yeast overgrowth in the gut as well. Just start slow and don't start downing MCT or you might get "the runs" (as in running to the bathroom).

A study published in *Lipids* even found that dietary supplementation of coconut oil actually reduced

abdominal fat. Healthy fats make you slim!
https://pubmed.ncbi.nlm.nih.gov/19437058/

Coconut is fun and easy to incorporate in so many recipes like smoothies. Coconut meat can be thrown on a salad. Coconut oil is great to use for extra flavor on veggies and in healthier treats. Dried coconut is a perfect addition to a homemade trail mix with dry roasted nuts.

Avocado Appreciation

Leading the charge of the healthy fat brigade are avocados. This wonder fruit is essentially Mother Nature's butter.

Avocados pack in healthy monounsaturated fats that contain oleic acid, which can actually help quiet feelings of hunger, according to a *Food Function* study. They also give you a nice amount of protein and fiber.

pubmed.ncbi.nlm.nih.gov/25347552

www.eatthis.com/high-fiber-foods

Avocados also give you tryptophan and magnesium for a great night's sleep. One whole avocado is packed with close to 30 grams!

Regan has found from experience that, when his dogs would eat avocados while he lived in Hawaii, their hair looked so much healthier. He also loves how it helps him to sleep better.

As for anyone who loves avocado toast, just cut the toast out and use the avocado to make so many delicious creations like guacamole, sliced on top of a burger or salad, add some sea salt and olive oil on top (more fat!), and you are golden.

My favorite dessert is chocolate avocado mousse made with stevia. You don't taste the avocado once blended with cacao and almond milk, you can top it with berries, sliced nuts, or coconut flakes, and it's creamy, rich, and delicious. No guilt, tons of great fat! I only use four ingredients, and there are many varieties now online!

What's the Buzz about Butter?

In 1961, Ancel Keys, a physiologist, claimed that saturated fat in the diet clogged arteries and caused heart disease.

It was this same information that influenced the diet of President Eisenhower who had a massive heart attack and Crohn's Disease. Ancel Keys wanted to find the cause of Eisenhower's heart attack and landed on saturated fats as the culprit.

Eisenhower was put on a very strict diet with no eggs and no saturated fats. He could have dry toast with a little bit of butter once a week. Despite the dietary changes, Eisenhower continued on a downward path with worsening health and increased cholesterol levels, but they kept him on the no saturated fat diet anyway. They replaced the saturated fat with vegetable oils.

It turns out, they were wrong. Fast forward to 2014, and you can read articles and see a *Time Magazine* cover titled "Eat Butter" where scientists reversed the narrative and stated saturated fats do not cause heart disease after all.

Why is butter good for you?

Above and beyond the satiating fat, it has Butyrate! We talked about Butyrate and how supportive it is to gut and colon health in the Gut chapter. Butyrate, a short chain saturated fatty acid, feeds your gut bacteria. It also protects against mental illness, increases energy expenditure and overall body composition, reduces the negative effects of Type I Diabetes, decreases intestinal permeability, and reduces inflammation!

Bad Fats

While you've now learned there are so many healthy fats to consume and gain benefits from, and even more than we have listed in this chapter, there are still fats you should avoid that can harm your health.

These include oils like sunflower oil, safflower oil, canola, corn, cottonseed, peanut, soy, and vegetable oils, margarine, artificial trans fat, and oils made from genetically modified grain.

> *"America's most widely consumed oil causes genetic changes in the brain: Soybean oil linked to metabolic and neurological changes in mice"*
> *~ScienceDaily.*
> www.sciencedaily.com/releases/2020/01/200117080827.htm

This just came out in 2020! It's more proof that widely overused, over-consumed bad oils are causing the brain and body serious harm.

Many of these oils have been denatured or processed to the point where they quickly go rancid. You'll find the majority of these oils in boxed and bagged processed junk foods like cookies, cakes, crackers, chips, dressings, sauces, and roasted nuts. I always tell my clients to only eat dry roasted or raw nuts to get the health benefits, and watch out for these oils in nut butters as well!

Always check your labels because if it says "roasted", there is most likely an oil added as listed above. Many brands also add sugar on top of the processed oil. Nuts and nut butters taste SO delicious on their own and do not need the junk additions!

You also want to be careful with dairy. If you do tolerate dairy, be sure to always buy organic and get full fat! Avoid skim, non-organic pasteurized conventional milk, cheese, cottage cheese, yogurts, or any products made from factory farming practices. As you've learned, they also inject them with growth hormones.

Dairy shows up in a lot of processed desserts as well, including powdered milk, condensed milk, and any ice cream that contains non-organic junk dairy. There are so many great organic clean dairy based ice creams and even non-dairy alternatives now, so you can still enjoy quality ice cream!

Drink milk and eat dairy that's full fat, from grass-fed cows, no growth hormones or antibiotics used (organic) and if you can tolerate it, raw dairy products are offered in certain stores and are delicious. I've had creamy delicious raw organic cheddar because, when I indulge in dairy on occasion, I only want the best. Conventional Kraft cheese that isn't even close to real cheese is just gross! Get the good stuff.

As you learned in the protein chapter, it's best to follow all those same guidelines when purchasing fattier meats, eggs, fish, etc.

Lastly, if you are cooking with healthy oils at higher temperatures, you want to go with avocado oil or coconut oil as they can withstand higher temperatures. Ghee is also a great alternative if you don't digest casein and lactose in butter well, as it's been boiled out of the ghee! Just make sure to steer clear of junk vegetable oils.

Ketones: An Alternative Source of Energy

Three ketones (chemicals made by the body) get activated when you start burning fats for fuel! This is called ketosis.

Those three ketones are acetoacetate, beta-hydroxybutyric acid, and acetone.

Turns out, your stem cells love ketones!

At MIT, Omer Yilmaz and colleagues fasted mice for 24 hours to study how the fasted state impacts intestinal stem cells. They found that a single fast augments intestinal stem cell function in both young and aged mice by boosting fat metabolism.

It appears that using fats for energy preserves the health and function of intestinal stem cells, and that the ability to break down and use fats for energy is impaired in older individuals, unless they fast.

news.mit.edu/2018/fasting-boosts-stem-cells-regenerative-capacity-0503

"Acute fasting regimens have pro-longevity and regenerative effects in diverse species, and they may represent a dietary approach to enhance aged stem cell activity in tissues."

Struggling Digesting Fats?

If you don't have a gallbladder you could benefit greatly from bile salts. Your gallbladder affects your ability to digest fats, and you still want to be able to get all the benefits of healthy fats in your diet.

The Food Pyramid

Remember this outdated model of eating where carbohydrates made up the majority of what was recommended for a healthy diet? Fast forward, and we've increased obesity, cardiovascular disease, and diabetes to epidemic levels. Imagine if we could go back in time and reverse it so healthy fats (then listed at the very top of the food pyramid, signifying to eat as little as possible) were a staple in everyone's diet.

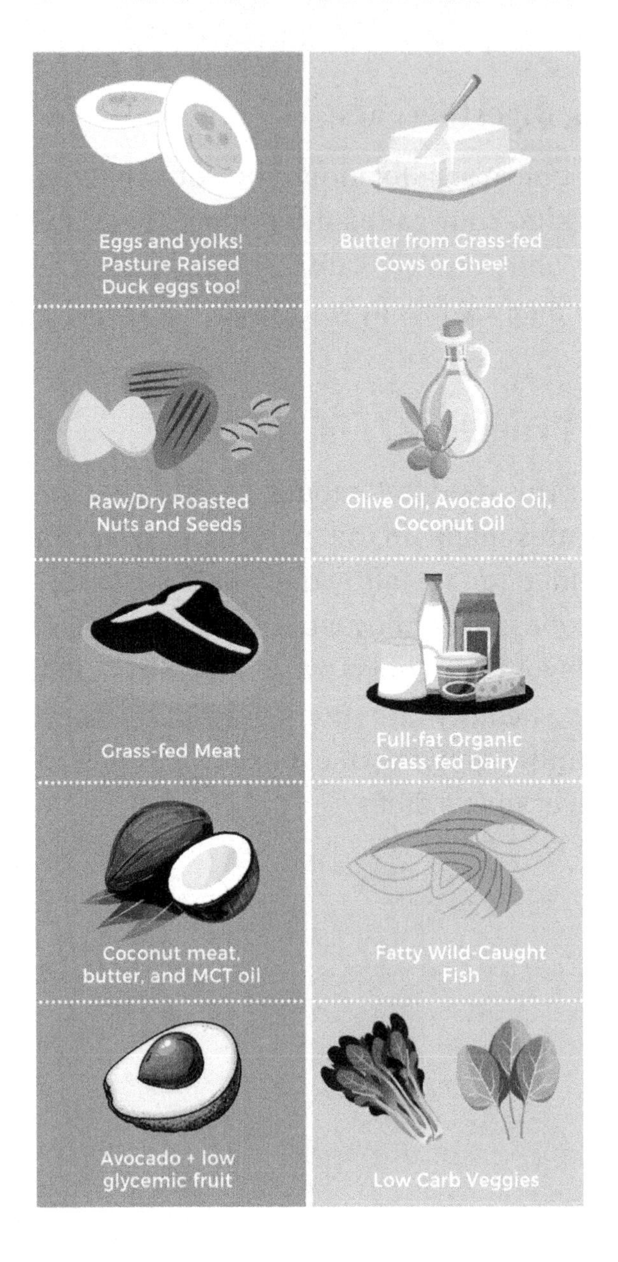
HIGH FAT
LOW CARB
Eggs and yolks!
Pasture Raised
Duck eggs too!
Butter from Grass-fed
Cows or Ghee!
Raw/Dry Roasted
Nuts and Seeds
Olive Oil, Avocado Oil,
Coconut Oil
Grass-fed Meat
Full-fat Organic
Grass fed Dairy
Coconut meat,
butter, and MCT oil
Fatty Wild-Caught
Fish
Avocado + low
glycemic fruit
Low Carb Veggies

What Does a High Fat, Low Carb Diet Look Like?

I don't know about you but thinking about all these healthy fats, and seeing those photos makes me want to eat! Time for your Challenge!

Challenge:

Add healthy fats into your diet. Aim for 120 grams per day if you are in good digestive health and don't have gallbladder issues. Use our recommended examples to add these superb foods into your diet and feel the huge difference in energy and vitality!

Peptide:

AOD-9604 for Optimizing Fat Metabolism

AOD-9604 is a great fat loss peptide that prevents lipogenesis (fat accumulation) and triggers lipolysis (fat burning) and helps you burn stubborn areas of fat as energy. In my clinical practice, I have seen patients lose an average of 10 pounds on this peptide, and studies show it can also help stabilize blood sugar. pubmed.ncbi.nlm.nih.gov/11146367

Using AOD-9604 in combination with either MOTS-c or 5-amino-1-MQ will maximize your results. This has been a breakthrough for many of my patients who have struggled to turn on metabolism.

Chapter Fifteen
The Barely Known Secret of Peptides to Expand Your Health

PEPTIDES

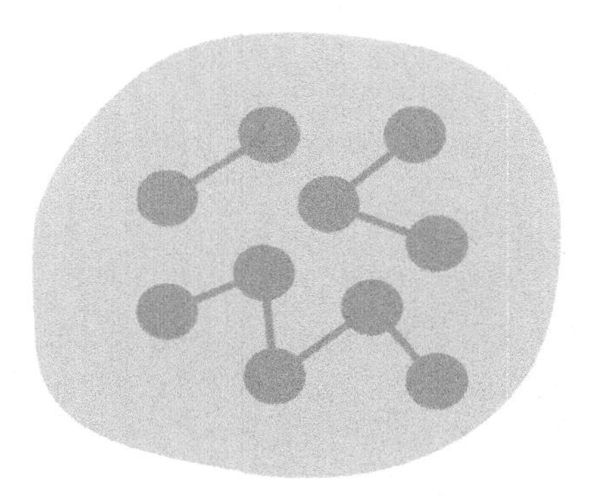

The Future of Medicine

Mindset Fourteen
Peptides can provide such a phenomenal upgrade to my health... in less time than other treatments out there.

"Peptides are naturally occurring biological molecules. Peptides are found in all living organisms and play a key role in all manner of biological activity. Like proteins, peptides are formed (synthesized) naturally from transcription of a sequence of the genetic code, DNA. Transcription is the biological process of copying a specific DNA gene sequence into a messenger molecule, mRNA, which then carries the code for a given peptide or protein. Reading from the mRNA, a chain of amino acids is joined together by peptide bonds to form a single molecule.

"There are 20 naturally occurring amino acids, and like letters into words, they can be combined into an immense variety of different molecules. When a molecule consists of two to 50 amino acids, it is called a peptide, whereas a larger chain of >50 amino acids generally is referred to as a protein."

Below is a compilation of the peptide suggestions per chapter in this book, and a brief description.

Keep in mind that each of these peptides does so many things for your health above and beyond what is listed! If you are interested in learning more, please contact us to schedule a consultation. We are also including our top recommendations for Peptide providers so that more patients can gain access to this wonderful innovative treatment option.

Peptide for Stress: Selank

- **Selank:** This peptide has been used in place of anxiety meds. It's great for eating disorders, food addictions, and can replace food as a healthy self soothing technique.
- Selank is a branch of amino acids that work by expressing the gene for the GABA neurotransmitter. www.frontiersin.org/articles/10.3389/fphar.2017.00089/full
- In a study of 60 patients with anxiety, Selank was found to improve the emotional health of the participants and had positive impacts on their quality of life that lasted beyond the duration of the study. https://pubmed.ncbi.nlm.nih.gov/25176261
- Selank is administered as a nasal spray and is one of the best peptides that I've found for relieving that feeling of angst that can derail me from enjoying life. My wife has commented on the calm that she notices with it as well. I have some patients who use it as needed and others who wish to stay on it long-term.
- Another added benefit of using Selank is that it also carries anti-viral properties. One study showed that the replication of the influenza virus was stopped with the use of Selank. It's ability to equalize TH1/TH2/Treg cytokine pathways directly and indirectly through the central nervous system with no known side effects make this a go-to with any concerns of viral infections including COVID-19.

Peptide for Respiratory Support: Thymosin Alpha 1

- **Thymosin Alpha 1:** Your Thymus gland shrinks as you age. Breathe deeper and support immunity, lungs, and cardiovascular system with this Peptide.
- You have an immune treasure next to your lungs called the Thymus gland. Every time you breathe, you stimulate blood flow for immune cell production. This gland trains your white blood cells, specifically, your T-lymphocytes, which are key defense cells for viral and other types of infection, to recognize threats. The thymus gland works through peptide pathways like thymosin alpha-1, Thymulin, Thymosin beta-4, or the actin binding potential-7 (APB-7) pathway.
- As we age our thymus gland shrinks which can leave our immune system with less intelligent capabilities to recognize and combat infections. www.endocrineweb.com/endocrinology/overview-thymus
- That's why using peptides like Thymulin-Zinc, Thymosin Alpha 1 or ABP-7 during times of immune stress can be helpful in training each of your new white blood cells in their duties of recognizing the threat and responding in a natural way. Researchers have found ways to bypass aging with the use of peptides that modulate enhanced immune intelligence. www.sciencedirect.com/science/article/abs/pii/089684119290152G

Peptides for Metabolism and Satiety: IGF-1/CJC1295/Ipamorelin

- **CJC1295:** This is what causes an increase in your pituitary to make growth hormone which helps your body feel more satiated when eating and energized.
- **Ipamorelin:** Somatostatin inhibitor that can tame ghrelin (the hormone that triggers food cravings). It increases the effectiveness of the growth hormone spike by seven times when used with CJC1295.
- **IGF-1:** Remember when you were a kid and could eat everything in sight and not gain a pound? That's because we have high levels of growth hormone as kids. The workhorse for Growth Hormone is IGF-1, and this is a peptide that can help diminish sugar cravings. IGF-1 receptors are 600 times more prevalent than insulin receptors in the body and is your number one fat burning hormone that stabilizes blood sugar spikes and drops. No more sugar cravings.
- CJC1295 is a peptide we use in conjunction with IGF-1 so that your pituitary makes more growth hormone so that your body feels more satiated when eating and energized. This peptide also helps you increase muscle mass.
- Ipamorelin helps balance out both growth hormone pathways in your pituitary gland. Its main function is to allow your body to express life giving

hormones by inhibiting Somatostatin. Ipamorelin tames ghrelin (the hormone that triggers food cravings), and it increases the effectiveness of the growth hormone spike by seven times when used with CJC1295.

Peptide for Pain Relief, Recovery, and Movement: TB4

- **Thymosin Beta 4:** Increases recovery post-workout, improves stem cell health in joints and connective tissue and skin, helps improve immunity, longevity, and energy.
- Have you ever been really sore after a workout? Maybe it's two or three days after you really pushed yourself, but the leg tightness and muscle aches are hard to forget.
- Thymosin Beta 4 is my go-to recovery peptide post workout. It improves stem cell health in joints, removes metabolic waste from muscles, and supports connective tissue, skin, and helps improve immunity. You can get a fragment of this made by my friend and colleague, Kent Holtorf, MD, called **TB4 FRAG** and see if it doesn't help.

Peptide for Sleep: DISP

- **DSIP:** Deep Sleep Inducing Peptides can retrain your pineal gland to express the right amount of melatonin at the right time. Sometimes, we DO need some help getting to and staying asleep. This is a sleep inducing peptide that induces delta brain waves. It works on the pineal gland to stabilize melatonin, serotonin, and oxytocin levels.

Peptide for Hydration: ARA-290

- Your kidneys are incredibly busy, and while **ARA-290** has been shown to stabilize blood sugar, Hemoglobin A1c levels, triglycerides, and cholesterol, it also works to promote erythropoietin, a hormone produced by the kidneys to produce red blood cells. pubmed.ncbi.nlm.nih.gov/25387363/
- I find that many patients who are chronically dehydrated also have anemic tendencies, kidney imbalances, and issues with cholesterol. ARA-290 is a lifesaver, and if you happen to have any neuropathy in your feet or your hands, studies show that this peptide helps heal the small nerve fibers that are damaged.

Peptide for Cold Therapy Circulation: Sarcotropin IPA

- **Sarcotropin IPA:** This one helps increase circulation, and specifically designed to build muscle mass and avoid muscle atrophy, stimulates the brain, and increases growth hormone without increasing appetite.
- Sarcotropin IPA is a peptide, amino acid and vitamin blend that has been shown to increase IGF-1 levels by 16%, improve muscle mass by nearly 10% and decrease visceral (organ) fat by 10% all in just three months. This popular formula has made it

through phase three clinical trials for Sarcopenia and is one of my favorites.

- Sarcotropin IPA helps increase circulation and is specifically designed to build muscle mass and avoid muscle atrophy. It also stimulates the brain and increases growth hormone without increasing appetite. It's a great aid in your cold exposure journey and is sure to maximize the health of your circulatory system.

Peptide for Timed Eating and Circadian Rhythm: Epitalon

- **Epitalon:** Reset circadian rhythms just like timed eating. This promotes longevity, decreases cholesterol, and improves cardiovascular health.
- This amazing peptide resets circadian rhythms just like timed eating. Epitalon is a natural occurring telomerase enzyme found in your pineal gland. Its expression promotes the length of the telomeres on the ends of your DNA which can result in greater stem cell activation and health.
- Research done by the Epitalon pioneer, Dr. Vladimir Khavinson shows that this peptide increases longevity by seven years, decreases cholesterol, and improves cardiovascular health, amongst many other physical and mental health benefits. Some studies are finding this peptide to be very effective in cancer prevention. [Khavinson, V.K., Bondarev, E., Butyugov, A.A. (2003). "Epithalon peptide induces telomerase activity and telomere

elongation in human somatic cells". *Bulletin of Experimental Biology and Medicine. 135*(6): 590–592]

Peptide for Liver and Hormonal Health: Tesamorelin

- **Tesamorelin** is 44 chained amino acids that have been studied extensively in diminishing belly fat and restoring normal liver enzyme production. This peptide has been incredibly helpful with my patients who have struggled to give up excessive alcohol consumption. They've remarked that they just don't like alcohol after using Tesamorelin, and they also see a decline in belly fat and an improvement in cognitive function.
- This peptide keeps your hypothalamus and pituitary glands turning out hormonal signals necessary for optimal health. It also signals your liver to metabolize those hormones so it can move on with aiding your body in digestion and detoxification.

Peptide for Gut Health: BPC-157

- **BPC-157:** Helps heal the endothelial cells damaged with leaky gut. Also helps with GERD (Gastrointestinal Reflux Disease), bloating, distention, food sensitivities, and many other digestive issues.
- Known as the "Wolverine" peptide, BPC-157 helps heal the endothelial cells damaged with leaky gut so that you can withstand any stressors thrown your

way. BPC-157 helps with GERD (Gastrointestinal Reflux Disease), EOE, bloating, distention, and a myriad of digestive issues.

- It's also known as the Wolverine peptide because of the way that it can assist in healing injuries to joints, tendons, and ligaments. In studies on rabbits it was shown to be effective for achilles tendon damage when compared with placebo. pubmed.ncbi.nlm.nih.gov/14554208/

Peptide for Veggies, blood sugar regulation, and metabolic support with carbohydrates: MOTS-c

- About a decade ago, researchers discovered the **MOTS-c** gene expression in Japanese people who lived beyond 100 years of age. www.ncbi.nlm.nih.gov/pmc/articles/PMC4693465
- Not only does MOTS-c promote longevity, in human and animal studies, it also helps with muscle growth, protects against insulin resistance, metabolism, heart, liver, and inflammation. MOTS-c mediates mitochondrial regulation of insulin sensitivity and metabolic homeostasis. It protects against age and diet-dependent insulin resistance and obesity.
- MOTS-c is the closest thing that researchers have found that mimics exercise and as this gene is expressed more in people who exercise. The use of this as a supplement to your program is a great idea.

Peptide for Digesting Protein and Leaky Gut: KPV

- **KPV** is a tri-peptide that naturally exists in your small intestine and its key role is calming inflammation. Studies show that in the presence of KPV, mice with colitis have a remission of symptoms. www.ncbi.nlm.nih.gov/pmc/articles/PMC5498804
- KPV can help eradicate any infections that may have come from improper digestion of your fats, proteins, or vegetables. It can also aid in eliminating Lyme disease, Epstein Barr virus or any chronic viral infections through the melano-corticoid system.

Peptide for Fat Digestion: AOD9604

- **AOD 9604** is a great fat loss peptide that prevents lipogenesis (fat accumulation) and triggers lipolysis (fat burning) and helps you burn stubborn areas of fat as energy. In my clinical practice, I have seen patients lose an average of 10 pounds on this peptide and studies show it can also help stabilize blood sugar. pubmed.ncbi.nlm.nih.gov/11146367/
- Using AOD 9604 in combination with either MOTS-c or 5-amino-1-MQ will maximize your results. This has been a breakthrough for many of my patients who have struggled to turn on metabolism.

Conclusion

You will love the boost you get from peptides, but make sure to get professional help with them. Ordering them from suspicious labs or online can be dangerous. Peptides made in selective compounding pharmacies are an investment but well worth the additional cost because you are getting the real thing. Reach out to me if you'd like to see if they can help you at regan@gowellness.com.

Chapter Sixteen
Are You Wasting Precious Time?

WASTING PRECIOUS TIME

Don't Just Guess: Test the 3, 4, 5 Method of Healing

When Regan and the Go Wellness Team sent me the book *Who Not How* by Dan Sullivan and Benjamin Hardy, I immediately realized the secret ingredient I had been leaving out of my life for SUCH a long time. Leaving out this one thing caused me to work harder, not smarter, feel greater stress, and unnecessarily waste precious time.

What was it? I was seeking to reach goals by doing everything myself, and when a challenge would arise, I would ask, "How am I going to get this done by myself without spending any money?"

Working hard and independently has taught me that I can do a LOT more than I ever thought possible, but I also spent so much more time, energy, and sometimes money unnecessarily in the process when I could have simply asked for help.

Working as a coach with some of the best doctors, NPs, NDs, DOs, nutritionists, and holistic healers in the country, if not the world, I would try to take some of their advice and immediately apply it on myself to see if it would work. Working so closely with them, I didn't feel comfortable admitting I was a health coach still struggling with my own health goals.

In my mind, I was supposed to be this perfect image of health in order to help others. My ego got in the way at every step, too ashamed to simply say, "Will you help me?" I was too scared I would be harshly judged by these amazing healers who walked the talk.

Now, to some degree, I still applaud self-exploration and experimentation, but this level of "do it yourself" thinking led me down a rabbit hole of trying so many different things without first understanding WHY I was feeling a certain way to begin with. Plus, getting trapped in cyclical patterned thinking didn't lead to answers. Your symptoms and diagnosis may be similar to mine, if not identical, but how we both got to feeling that way is usually very different.

Some people develop thyroid conditions from heavy metal toxicity. Some develop it from blood sugar irregularity. Some develop it from the foods they are eating, not realizing they are causing massive inflammation and internal harm.

How you course-correct the thyroid based on those three examples can be a bit different for each scenario. It's not 1 + 1 = 2 for every patient with the same condition. Regan and his team are the best of the best and can take you through a comprehensive functional blood chemistry test and determine exactly what you need. Don't be scared to ask for help at regan@gowellness.com.

For years, I was trying different dietary protocols, cutting tons of things out, and trying supplements I thought would completely transform my life. What I was left with was a lot of money spent and no clearer answers/resolutions to the problems plaguing me. I convinced myself for years that tests were not my answer, so I'd avoid them, or I would try something, receive a negative result, and feel downtrodden.

One of your best health investments is to get functional medicine blood work done once or twice a year.

I wasn't getting the clear-cut answers I so desperately wanted to hear, which went something like this: "Anne, we finally know the root cause of all your surface symptoms. This is exactly what you need to do and you are guaranteed to feel 100% better if you do it!"

Healing, I have learned, doesn't look nor sound that way. Even if you do have access to some of the best of the best providers. It's a winding journey filled with ups and downs and twists and turns, victories, and even dark holes, yet that's not meant to deter anyone on the ride.

In my journey, I've realized that, in trying to cherry-pick my way to wellness all by myself, I was missing the bigger picture. I am not meant to heal myself alone on this journey. If my mindset is what currently led me to where I am now, how on earth am I to get myself to change when the behaviors are following the leadership of my own rigid belief system? Sometimes, you need outer perspective.

To get better, we need a "Who", not another "How". I'm telling you this so that you stop trying so hard to do it alone. If tears are welling up right now, welcome them. You've probably suffered a long time in silence, trying so hard for so long to "figure it out".

Asking for help from experts who are already where you want to be, and who have already accomplished getting others just like you where you want to be is a much greater solution, one that will save you countless hours, tons of money, and emotional suffering trying to piece it together yourself with Amazon-purchased supplements, diet books, and good intentions.

If you are still going to a traditional doctor's office that calls out minimal markers simply because your insurance will cover it, but your doctor doesn't explain what those markers are and why they are important, or what the optimal levels are within a reference range, you are going to the wrong provider.

If your provider doesn't make time to answer all your questions (within reason) during your visit and shuffles you out the door after a five-minute lab review where you are told "your labs look fine" yet you feel like utter crap, or you are given a prescription without any other support for how to correct your health concerns, you are going to the wrong provider.

Is my frustration coming out? Yes. I've experienced this first-hand, and it's one of the reasons I became a health coach for doctors who KNOW the importance of diet and lifestyle. There are doctors and providers who give their patients the time, care, and attention they deserve to truly be educated on how the body works and what's truly possible.

I love a provider who says, "I'm going to teach you how your body works, how things went wrong, and what you can do about it so you feel in control of your health and are not dependent on me, a medication, or a surgery to get well and stay well." Sign me up! That's the doctor I want to work with.

In finding the right "Who" to be my teammate and help me decipher and uncover what was really going on, I could have saved myself a lot of time and frustration trying to do it alone. Hence the importance of receiving accountability, support, and guidance on your own health and healing journey.

Above and beyond not making my mistake of avoiding asking for help, I'd like to also stress the importance of testing without guessing your way to optimal wellbeing.

Why Test?

I've convinced myself over the years that receiving a needed test result that did look normal was a failure. On the contrary, as Dr. Dan Kellams taught me, any answer, either positive or negative, is one step closer to knowing the truth. Without it, we continue guessing what *may* be going right or wrong within our system, and that can lead us down a very wrong path in trying to solve it. I did this thinking for years I had yeast overgrowth without ever actually doing a stool test.

Dr. Dan, who works with Regan as the Go Wellness creative director, once brilliantly explained how he imparts the importance of lab tests to his patients. When a patient asked, "Why do I need to test for things like Vitamin D when I'm physically in pain? Why is that, of all things, important?" Dan replied, "Do you know what a Vitamin D deficiency feels like?" "No." "Neither do I. That's why it's so important to test it," and yes, Vitamin D does support so many pathways that it can influence your immune health, your body's ability to heal, and pain/inflammation.

So many times, we want to feel the immediate ROI from supplements, but the body is a complex work of art. If you studied how each individual micronutrient and macronutrient works on the deepest, cellular level, it would blow your mind.

Did you know that bacteria can enter your bones and further perpetuate issues like arthritis? Pain and bacteria are related?? Yes.

Did you know that Vitamin D is one of the most important hormones (Yes, it's a hormone, not a vitamin) that can impact everything from your brain health to bone health, to mood, to a cascade of other illnesses if not in optimal range? So many people are walking around not knowing just how low their Vitamin D levels are without the proper testing and assessment, and how that, if ameliorated, could tremendously impact their health.

Did you know that "reference ranges" provided on labs are different depending on where you live in the world? It's not based on what is optimal but rather, a generic range for the population you live within. My Vitamin D levels were just on the cusp of being deficient by generic standards for years, but because they weren't drastically low to the point of causing rickets, my previous doctors never stressed the importance to me of taking Vitamin D. I lived in the Midwest and East Coast for the first 30 years of my life. Now that I know the importance, I take it every single day. Do I still seek sunlight? Absolutely, but I love knowing exactly what I'm taking in and seeing my labs climb.

It's important for me to impart what it means to have your labs fully explained to you so that you can feel empowered as a patient and make the best choices possible. It's meant to help you feel hopeful, and not helpless, believing your only chance of feeling better is medication or surgery, and your only option is to "manage" the symptoms you have rather than seeking to understand and eliminate them at the root cause.

Think of it like a tree or a plant. If your tree or plant is dying, and you are wanting it to thrive, I would think you'd assess what the cause might be. Is it not getting enough water? Is it getting enough nutrients in the soil? Does it get enough sunlight each day? Is it the time of year for it to shed? You'd assess the environmental factors and fundamentals of what a plant needs to grow and thrive. Why don't we treat ourselves the same way?

If you have gas and irritable bowel syndrome, do you look at your diet and lifestyle, or simply laugh it off, masking the symptoms of discomfort with gas jokes, and go on about your usual routine? Do you just run to the bathroom when no one is looking?

When you feel tired, do you ask, "Am I thirsty right now? Did I hydrate enough today and get adequate sleep?" Maybe you simply say, "Ah, well, it must be time to eat again," without stopping to think about what your body might truly need.

I'm asking you to question the beliefs and unconscious patterns that have led you to where you are, bringing greater awareness and therefore greater success to your life.

This is why Regan and his team always take patients through the "3 Ts" to greater health and wellbeing, which is a part of their 3-4-5 method to patient success.

The first T stands for Testing. The second T stands for Treating. The third T is for Teaching. They want to gather data first without blindly making recommendations, potentially wasting your time and money. They want to use that data to inform every single decision so that every treatment is customized and selected to get the best outcomes. They also want to teach you to understand how your body works and why they are choosing a particular path of care so that you feel 100% clear with your plan, guaranteed.

We can't exercise, eat, breathe, sleep, or do cold showers for you. This book was meant to be a mechanism for health independence, education, and transformation in your day-to-day life. However, it is also meant as a stepping stone to receiving the ultimate care you deserve with a team of healthcare providers who care deeply and want the best for you. You get access to some of the most cutting edge science and research in peptide therapy, nutrition, and fitness, along with a powerful, loving community.

If this resonates with you, is it a ridiculous idea for me to ask you regan@gowellness.com right now to call a functional medicine provider or email Regan at, and ask for help with your health concerns? I wish someone had sat me down and told me all of this much, much sooner.

Therefore, I felt the need to share in hopes it inspires you to know you are not alone, you are not meant to walk on your health journey alone, and they are here for you every step of the way.

It's been an honor and a pleasure to co-author this book with Regan's unique genius, and to share many stories and tips that I love in hopes it makes your life 1% better every single day.

Don't forget, for purchasing this book, you receive access to join the live Group Coaching HAC community. If you thought this was jam packed, can you believe that we've created five additional themed HAC courses and continue creating more? We've taught our patients how to revitalize their brain health, heart health, energy, thyroid health, immune function, burn fat like a boss and we keep going strong. Why? We never stop healing.

Call to Action

- Join HACs online and get a consultation with the team at www.acueastwest.com/contact-us
- Go to thesmartmedicine.com for guidance on nootropics, supplements and peptides.

This book is not intended as a substitute for the medical advice of physicians. The reader should consult a physician in matters relating to his/her health and particularly with respect to any symptoms that may require diagnosis or medical attention.